Dr. Nash's
Natural Diet Book

by David T. Nash, M.D.

GROSSET & DUNLAP
A FILMWAYS COMPANY
Publishers • New York

Individual achievements gratify the ego, but the truth is that most worthwhile efforts require the convergence of many skills. So it is with this book.

Sheila Crowley edited the manuscript with consummate skill and a singleness of purpose. Dr. M. MacLaren infused in me an interest in mythology that brought the tales of the ancients to life with startling reality. Helene Shirer provided much of the research material, and Celia Adelphi and Joan Rogus contributed to the nutritional information in the manuscript. Beth Caspin, Lillian Cohn, Joanne Dennis and Linda Landaw reviewed some of the earlier material, and Helene Wallace helped in the myriad of administrative details. Concetta Corasaniti prepared multiple versions of the manuscript. Sue Martin supervised part of the research program. Special thanks are due to Aunt Sadie Bettigole, Helen Naimark and Joseph Gorgoni for their tasty contributions to the recipes in this book.

Finally, I must acknowledge those volunteers and patients who followed the diet and made it possible for others to follow and succeed on the Natural Diet.

Copyright © 1978 by David T. Nash, M.D.
All rights reserved
Published simultaneously in Canada
Library of Congress catalog card number: 77-78343
ISBN 0-448-14647-9
Printed in the United States of America
1978 Printing

To my mother, who made my life possible
To my wife, who made it meaningful

Contents

1.

Thin Is a Matter of Choice

"I stuffed myself and still lost weight."
—Emergency-room nurse on the Natural Diet

We all want to be thin! If wanting made it so, none of us would be fat. Of course, we also all like to eat—at least I do. On traditional diets, this can be a terrific problem. Amazing as it may seem, however, you *can* have your cake and eat it too. The Natural Diet, based as it is on good, sound nutrition, makes this possible.

No specters of starvation and self-denial need appear to frighten you away from this diet. On the Natural Diet, you can eat until you are full. You can eat out. You can eat grits, corn on the cob, curried rice, or tortillas. Foods like bread, potatoes, spaghetti, and bagels are not *verboten*. In fact, they are the foundation of this diet!

Are you hungry yet? Most people I see who have tried dieting were either hungry or felt deprived. On the Natural Diet they all felt they were getting enough to eat. Many complained that there was too much food at breakfast and lunch! None felt ill, faint, or weak. In fact, many of the volunteers who tested the diet said that they felt better than they had in years. Some of these people work, some have families, some entertain, and most had failed on other diets.

The Natural Diet is a wise diet. It has evolved from the most recent nutritional research. It has been tested experimentally and has some beneficial side effects. It will lower the fats in your blood as well as your chances of having a heart attack or a stroke! This bold statement is supported by solid documentation. A group of hospital employees who were carefully studied while on the diet demonstrated significant reductions of the fats in their blood. Other studies have linked the progression of hardening of the arteries to the amount of fats in the blood.

This diet, based primarily on cereal grains, will help you achieve more than simple weight loss. It will help reduce your cholesterol intake as well as your chances of developing high blood pressure and diabetes. It will also help reduce your food budget, since cereal grains are less expensive than most meats or cheeses. It will provide all the vitamins and minerals you need. It is a safe, sane, complete diet.

Both what you eat and how much you eat are important if you are on a diet. Your weight is determined by how much you eat compared to how much you burn for energy. Whenever you eat more than you need for energy, body repairs, and new muscle growth, you accumulate fat.

You can learn to tip the scales in the other direction. This diet uses food exchanges, suggesting roughly equivalent energy-value foods that can be substituted for each other. Your calorie-counting is done for you, and you really can have almost anything to eat. The exchange system helps you choose wisely by presenting food alternatives in the precise amounts that will promote weight loss. For example, hard cheeses may be substituted for the same amount of meat, and an ounce of Scotch can fill in for a cereal allotment. This concept will become clearer as you read on.

Now the catch: You must decide to eat less meat. Ounce for ounce, a lean steak has many more calories than a baked potato. Even lean meat contains more calories of fat than of protein. Since it is high in animal fat, meat is high in cholesterol; and cholesterol contributes to heart disease. The trick, obviously, is to lower your intake of animal fat; the Natural Diet shows you how.

Have you decided that it is time to diet? Well, if you are not sure, check the table in this chapter which lists ideal weights. You may be surprised to find that your ideal weight is lower than you would have wished. This is because the concept of *ideal* weight is not the same as *average* weight. We are dealing with ideal weight because that is the weight at which you'll look best and probably live longest.

Not everyone who wants to lose weight is really obese. Lots of people just want to lose ten or twenty pounds of excess baggage. Also, many people who have lost a lot of weight find losing the last few pounds is the hardest. Let me give you an example of two women, each five feet two inches tall and thirty years old. One weighs 170 pounds; the other weighs 120 pounds. The ideal weight for both might be 110 pounds. The heavier woman will have considerably less difficulty going from 170 pounds to 160 pounds than the lighter one will have going from 120 to 110 pounds. Why? For a variety of reasons that are important to understand before you attempt any diet.

IDEAL WEIGHTS FOR MEN AND WOMEN

According to Height and Frame. Ages 25 and Over

Height (In Shoes)	Weight in Pounds (In Indoor Clothing)		
	Small Frame	Medium Frame	Large Frame
Men			
5' 2"	112−120	118−129	126−141
3"	115−123	121−133	129−144
4"	118−126	124−136	132−148
5"	121−129	127−139	135−152
6"	124−133	130−143	138−156
7"	128−137	134−147	142−161
8"	132−141	138−152	147−166
9"	136−145	142−156	151−170
10"	140−150	146−160	155−174
11"	144−154	150−165	159−179
6' 0"	148−158	154−170	164−184
1"	152−162	158−175	168−189
2"	156−167	162−180	173−194
3"	160−171	167−185	178−199
4"	164−175	172−190	182−204
Women			
4' 10"	92− 98	96−107	104−119
11"	94−101	98−110	106−122
5' 0"	96−104	101−113	109−125
1"	99−107	104−116	112−128
2"	102−110	107−119	115−131
3"	105−113	110−122	118−134
4"	108−116	113−126	121−138
5"	111−119	116−130	125−142
6"	114−123	120−135	129−146
7"	118−127	124−139	133−150
8"	122−131	128−143	137−154
9"	126−135	132−147	141−158
10"	130−140	136−151	145−163
11"	134−144	140−155	149−168
6' 0"	138−148	144−159	153−173

Courtesy of Metropolitan Life Insurance Company. Derived primarily from data of the *Build and Blood Pressure Study, 1959*, Society of Actuaries.

We all hear a lot about water retention, which is a most important factor in weight loss. Misunderstanding this factor can seriously handicap your dieting efforts. *The heavier you are in relation to your ideal weight, the more fluid your body will retain.* Excess fluid can be mobilized far more readily than excess fat or muscle, which means it can be got rid of much more quickly. This is the phenomenon that underlies the claims of diet faddists who proclaim a "ten-pound weight loss in a weekend" or "lose forty pounds with no effort in twenty days." Baloney! It takes effort to lose forty pounds of *flesh*, and you may as well adjust to this fact of life. Losing ten pounds of *fluid* over a weekend is fine, but what of the next ten? And what about the 120-pound woman, who does not have ten pounds of fluid to lose? If she did lose ten pounds of fluid, it would be solely because of *dehydration*. Dehydration is what we do to potatoes to make them fit into a smaller box. Dehydrated foods were the way GIs were fed in World War II. The foods didn't taste very good, but they did occupy less space. Similarly, you won't feel very well dehydrated, even if you succeed in fooling the scale temporarily. You'll note that I say "temporarily"—that's because you'll probably regain almost all the lost weight the next time you drink fluids. And while you may occupy less space, you'll still have all the fat you started with.

The problem with fad diets is that they are almost never nutritionally balanced. Your body requires adequate fluid, vitamins, protein, carbohydrates, fats, fiber, bulk, and minerals for optimal health. So, on one of those fad diets, you feel—and really are—deprived of the essentials for good health. This is the reason it's so hard to *keep* off the weight you get off—your body begins to crave what it lacks, temptation sets in, and goodbye weight loss! Your body needs those missing nutrients for your general good health.

Most adults will not maintain their ideal weight after the age of thirty without some effort. Of course, we all know (and hate) the rare exception. Everyone has a friend who eats a lot and yet remains thin. This book is not intended for the occasional Twiggy. Such ectomorphs (long, thin people who never gain weight) often complain that they cannot gain weight. It's hard to be sympathetic.

Timing is important to dieting. When you start and how you feel when you start are very important to the rapidity of your weight loss. Most women retain salt and water just prior to their menstrual periods. Salt and water retention cause a deceptive weight gain. It is temporary and can be safely ignored.

People of either sex will find it hard to lose weight when they are suffering from emotional upset. The reasons are multiple: Depression results in a reduction of physical activity. Sex drive is diminished. The lack of other gratifications associated with depression often results in more eating to "reward" oneself in a misdirected effort to feel stronger or happier. Any severe emotional upset may result in a change in your eating pattern. While some people lose their appetites and eat less, most people with weight problems react to stress by eating more.

The mere idea of dieting is enough to depress some people. Some diets are grim. The Natural Diet is different—it is evolutionary, not revolutionary. It also works.

Mr. R. P., a sixty-year-old truck driver, lost twenty pounds and gained normal blood pressure. In the beginning he had some difficulty choosing among the alternative foods allowed on the Natural Diet. In the end the ranges of food choices sustained him. After three months he needed new clothes! Mr. R. P., now a size 36 waist, will never wear his size 42 pants again. Incidentally, Mr. R. P. confesses that he did and does occasionally reward himself with a little indiscretion—"like a few beers."

Believe it! Look at the possibilities: Here are a few samples of the choices you can make about your own meals. You'll see what I mean about variety. (Remember to use no sugar or cream with coffee or tea.)

Breakfast

¼ fresh melon

2 cups of dry cereal (Puffed Wheat or Rice)

or 1 cup of cooked cereal

or 2 slices of toast

1 cup of skim milk

coffee or tea

Lunch

a tuna fish sandwich on pumpernickel bread

or a ham sandwich on a hard roll

or a lean roast beef sandwich on rye bread

or 2 slices of smoked salmon on a bagel

or 1 cup of cooked spaghetti with a stewed tomato sauce

or a turkey sandwich with lettuce and mayonnaise

a tossed salad

or a serving of broccoli

or a serving of cauliflower

or lettuce and tomatoes

or dill pickles

or a cup of vegetable soup

an orange, apple, or pear

or ⅓ cup of fresh pineapple

coffee, tea, or low-calorie soft drink

Dinner

4 ounces of roast chicken
or 3 ounces of ham
or 4 ounces of turkey
or 3 ounces of hamburger, lean
or 3 ounces of beef
or 3 ounces of veal
or 5 ounces of fish

succotash with ½ cup lima beans and ⅓ cup corn

tossed salad with low-calorie dressing

fresh or frozen blueberries

coffee or tea

Snack

1 cup of buttermilk

1 cup of popcorn
or 1 ounce of low-fat cheese
or 2 Rye Crisp crackers
or 1 ounce of cognac or brandy to sip during the evening

It might seem at first that the Natural Diet is excessively liberal. Indeed, many people on it worried that they'd be eating too much. In fact, 96 percent of the volunteers lost weight on it—and so will you. With a minimum of effort at menu planning, you should enjoy this diet and learn something about proper serving sizes of food and about nutrition. This information is essential to successful dieting.

Many people experience a number of uncomfortable symptoms on quickie diets because they are following a nutritionally deficient regime. This diet is different. You should experience no deficiency symptoms because the diet has been designed to meet all your nutritional needs. You'll feel better on this diet than you felt before, on or off other diets, and as you begin to lose weight, you'll get the kind of reinforcement you need to continue dieting. This diet succeeds without deceptive water shifts.

Before going into the specifics of the Natural Diet, I would like to mention a few simple aids. Modifying your behavior will help you stick to the diet and make it more comfortable for you. The best help for any dieter is a diet diary—a diary in which you simply record what you eat and when you eat it. By keeping such a record, you will begin to learn your pattern of indulgence and how to master it. Chapter 3 discusses the specifics of keeping such a diary. When you feel the need to eat between meals, look for physical diversion. Plan an evening tennis game, go swimming, or take a long walk to avoid temptation. You will derive other benefits as well, since exercise is another component of successful dieting.

There are definite ways to make dieting easier. If you enjoy sweets, try to eat the fruit serving allotted to each meal first; this will often satisfy your appetite earlier in the meal. Plan to eat slowly enough to let a sense of fullness register before you finish the meal (it takes about twenty minutes for your brain to send your stomach the message that you've had enough). Put the lower-calorie snacks in the front of your refrigerator and pantry; you'll see them first. You can avoid tempting, high-calorie food by not purchasing any and by placing those already in the house in inconvenient places, like the back of closets.

Another way of enjoying your diet and making it easier is to make low-calorie dishes more attractive with garnishes, spices, and condiments. If you plan your menu ahead of time, it will be easier for you to pay attention to what you eat. You'll be able to prepare only what you wish to eat—nothing more. Having regular mealtimes and a specific place to eat both help establish long-range food habits. People who modify their eating habits are more likely to maintain their ideal weight over the years.

Are you ready to begin a lifetime approach to staying thin and healthy the rest of your life? If so—read on: the best is yet to come.

2.

Getting Started

Tell me what you eat, and I will tell you what you are.
—Brillat-Savarin

One of the basics of the Natural Diet is the diet or meal plan. A diet plan is like a game plan. All games have rules, and dieting is no exception.

There are two cardinal rules in the diet game: The first is to *make a firm commitment* to diet, and the second is to *follow the meal plan,* which appears later in this chapter, closely. These two rules guarantee success. Once you recognize the advantages of the Natural Diet and integrate it into your life-style, you will see that it is actually quite easy to lose weight.

Plan on retaining your new eating habits for the rest of your life. You will not experience hunger pains, nor will you starve; instead, you will find that you can lose weight while eating a considerable amount of food.

There are several habits that can be self-defeating when you diet; avoid these right from the start. Do not skip meals; it is a false caloric economy. Many obese people suffer from the nighttime eating syndrome. They skip breakfast, eat a diminutive lunch and a large dinner. After dinner they eat, and they eat, and they eat. They often eat as much food *after* a complete dinner as they need for a whole day and evening. It is little wonder they experience insomnia, a "too full" feeling, and awaken the next day only to repeat the cycle, starting without breakfast. By nightfall they feel hungry; virtuous for having fasted all day, they resume eating as a well-earned "reward."

PORTION SIZES

Consider the portion size of anything you eat. A *serving* may mean different quantities for fruits, vegetables, cereals, and meats. You might eat three ounces of meat but eight ounces of vegetable, and call each a *portion*. It is a good idea to refer to the meal plan frequently, which tells you how much of what you should eat, until you know it by heart. Remember that if the recommended meat portion is one ounce and your limit is five ounces a day, then you are only fooling yourself when you consider your twelve-ounce steak a "serving."

Another habit to break is eating to reward yourself. Additional food cannot compensate you for a hard day. Your parents may have initiated the food-reward cycle, but as an adult you will have to find less self-defeating escapes. A brisk walk, exercise, reading a good diet book, sex, a shower, or going to bed early are all satisfactory alternatives (not necessarily in that order of preference).

Plan on developing good habits. If you know what constitutes an equivalent exchange for your favorite meal, it will make the diet easier to follow (this exchange system is explained more fully later on). It releases you from the obligation of counting calories. The Natural Diet includes a variety of attractively prepared foods and regular meals at appropriate times. You'll find recipes for a great many delicious meals at the back of this book. Food should delight the eye and fuel the body.

The Natural Diet involves changing many of your eating habits. You will modify and improve your eating behavior by eating the food choices and quantities allowed at each meal according to the meal plan. Don't force yourself to eat just to conform rigidly to the diet. However, you will come to enjoy the more full and complete breakfast this diet outlines. The dinner meal contains significantly less meat than most people eat. You cannot and should not add to the dinner meal by robbing your breakfast and lunch. If you make excessive modifications in the diet, you will sooner or later wind up with no diet at all and be back to your old eating patterns. It should be obvious to you by this time that the no-breakfast or no-lunch approach to dieting is not successful. If you follow it, this plan *will* work, so relax—you will soon see the benefits of the Natural Diet.

When you are home and it is convenient, weigh or measure the foods that you eat. Using a simple kitchen scale, this is not as difficult as it sounds. Without the scale you can still estimate the sizes of meat portions by their dimensions. Try a simple trick: Buy a pound of hamburger and divide it into four equal rectangles about one-half to five-eighths of an inch thick. Thereafter it will be quite simple for you to estimate what constitutes four ounces of uncooked meat or fish. Although an approximation, it is quite adequate for your purpose.

Liquids and vegetables are easily approximated by volume. Most fruit will provide no challenge to your skill in guessing the amount. We all can tell what a single apple, banana, or orange is, and with any kind of practice most of us can estimate a cup of strawberries. If you can accurately estimate servings, it will be easier for you to keep an accurate diet diary. Because you will know how much you are eating, you can enjoy a lifetime of good eating, while maintaining your health and proper weight.

MEALS

Plan on eating at regular times—times that are convenient for you and your family. When you eat breakfast and lunch is almost always determined by the realities of personal work loads and family, employment, school, business, or professional responsibilities. The one area that is quite flexible is the dinner hour and the time for the snack. You can develop a sensible pattern without undue manipulation of your life-style. Cutting down on late-night meals becomes possible only after you become aware of your eating patterns through the use of a diet diary, and resolve to correct them.

The snack is the meal that is most flexible and can most easily be modified to suit you. Evening snacks are the most common cause of dietary lapses. If you must munch, stick to celery, radishes, cucumbers, or carrots. A special low-calorie snack can be strawberries. Their cost may be prohibitive in winter, but they will do the trick when you need something sweet. Another trick is to cut up lettuce and top it with a low-calorie dressing. Several excellent ones are now available. For example, a low-calorie blue cheese dressing on the market contains only ten calories per teaspoon and consists largely of low-fat milk, buttermilk, corn syrup solids, and blue cheese bits.

Avoid making your menu very different from the rest of your family's. The Natural Diet is designed so that you do not have to deviate markedly from everyone else at home. What you will be doing is reducing the amount of meat you eat and supplementing your dinner with bread or a starchy vegetable.

HINTS FOR SUCCESSFUL DIETING

Plan on eating in a specific place, for example, the kitchen or the dining room; then avoid eating anywhere else. Do not eat while watching TV or reading a novel, since eating should be clearly defined as an interruption in your other activities. If you eat while you are doing something else, you usually eat more. Make the eating situation a complete activity in its own location. Plan on eating with someone else, if possible. Select what you are going to eat before the meal; leave the table when you are finished; and throw away the food scraps and leftovers that aren't enough for another meal.

This last point is important and deserves elaboration. We were all raised in a society which discourages waste; many people are offended by the concept of discarding food. I am sure you remember your parents admonishing you to clean your plate. Large posters in military food messes proclaim, "Take what you want, but eat what you take." Now I am asking you to throw away perfectly good food! Why? Because it is impossible to predict exactly how much you want—portions often exceed needs. During a meal, we may feel full and still have some food on our plate. Most of us will finish the remaining meat, potatoes, and dessert left on our plate—not because we crave it, not because we need it, not because we want it, but *only* because it is there! Learn to eat only as much as you really enjoy, then stop, even if food remains. Divorce yourself from the notion that you help a hungry person in a starving, overpopulated, underdeveloped third-world country by eating everything on your plate. All you do is add to your own girth. After you have thrown away a bit of food here and there, you will find that your ability to judge adequate serving sizes is improved. Eventually you will choose, buy, and serve smaller portions of food. If you feel guilty about throwing out these small amounts of food, remind yourself that when enough people follow the Natural Diet, less meat will be consumed and more cereal previously fed to cattle will become available to the world.

Good nutrition includes servings from all four food groups: meat, milk, cereals, and fruits and vegetables. Combining food from all groups provides better balanced and more interesting meals. Use the equivalents listed in the food groups in this chapter in planning your menus. These lists present foods that are equal in nutritional and caloric value; therefore, they can be substituted for one another. The lists will tell you the proper amounts. So if you're not in the mood for one food item, pick another that will satisfy you more. The Natural Diet uses this exchange system because it provides choices in every food category. You will be able to choose foods for convenience, economy, and appropriateness to your own needs and yet stick to the basic Natural Diet meal plan.

By following the Natural Diet you will learn how to exchange equivalent servings of one food for another. The diet provides a large variety of choices of approximately equal calories and specifies equivalent amounts. This puts both the responsibility and the freedom of choice squarely on your shoulders. Because you will make choices, you will and should begin to learn more about food equivalents and what foods are necessary daily. Following these suggestions will provide you with pleasure as well as nutrition.

The following pages list verbatim the instructions, meal plan, and food-group lists that have been used successfully by many dieters. You will probably wish to refer to the lists often as you continue reading about the diet. Frequent use of this material in the early stages of your diet will be helpful.

GENERAL DIET INSTRUCTIONS

1. Follow the meal plan exactly. Don't carry over foods allowed from one meal to the next. Eat *all* the foods allowed at each meal.
2. Weigh and measure foods when eating at home.
3. Eat at regular times each day.
4. Record daily all foods eaten and the quantity consumed (diet diary).
5. Eat slowly and chew food thoroughly.
6. Try to avoid a menu that is different from that of the rest of the family.
7. Develop an interest in a hobby or sport to take your thoughts off food.

MEAL PLAN

Meal	Food Group	Servings
Breakfast	Fruit	1
	Breads and cereals	2
	Milk, skim	1 cup
Lunch	Meat	2 oz.
	Bread and starch	2
	A vegetable	as desired
	Fat	1
	Fruit	1
Dinner	Meat	3 oz. or 4 oz. fowl, or 5 oz. fish
	Bread and starch	2
	A vegetable	as desired
	Fat	1
	Fruit	1
Snack	Milk, skim	1 cup
	Bread and starch	1

FOOD GROUPS

MILK

Any one of the following equals a one-cup serving:

Buttermilk made from skim milk	1 cup
Cottage cheese	2 ounces
Dry powdered skim milk	⅓ cup reconstituted to 1 cup liquid
Evaporated skim milk	½ cup undiluted

Skim milk or 99 percent fat-free milk	1 cup
Yogurt made from skim milk	1 cup

Avoid the following:

Commercial whipped toppings	Dried whole milk
Condensed milk	Evaporated whole milk
Cream (sweet or sour)	Ice cream and ice milk
Cream substitutes	Whole milk
	Whole-milk drinks

FATS AND OILS

Any one of the following equals one serving:

Avocado	⅛ of a ½-in.-thick slice (4 in. dia.)
Commercial salad dressings (must not contain sour cream)	1 Tbs.
Nuts (no coconut)	1 Tbs.
Olives	5 small
Peanut butter	2 tsp.
Specially prepared margarines	1 tsp.
Vegetable oil (corn oil, safflower oil, cottonseed oil, sunflower oil, and soybean oil are acceptable)	1 tsp.

Note: Margarine should be made from one of the allowed oils listed above. *Liquid*—not hardened, partially hardened, or hydrogenated—oil should be the first, therefore major, listed ingredient.

The meal plan includes a serving of fat or oil at breakfast, lunch, and dinner. At breakfast and lunch it might be best to use a specially prepared margarine, preferably one of the diet varieties, which have fewer calories per serving. They contain polyunsaturated fats and have little or no cholesterol, and are enriched with the fat-soluble vitamins A and D. Diet salad dressings, nuts, or a small portion of avocado may be used as the diet fat serving. It is wise to avoid butter, sour cream, and coconut, since they contain saturated fats. On occasion, hard cheeses may be substituted ounce for ounce for the meat serving, which also will contain the equivalent of one serving of fat. Some special low-cholesterol cheeses are made with corn oil, and each serving includes a fat equivalent.

The most important element of the Natural Diet is flexibility. You may find that on most days margarine is your chosen fat, but on other days you may want a handful of nuts. Put diet margarine on your popcorn; put some olives in your martini snack.

Consider the newly developed low-cholesterol eggs. Some of these have substantial amounts of fats and oils in them. When you intend to substitute low-cholesterol eggs for the breakfast cereal serving, remember that the fat and oil serving is included in the eggs. It might also be useful to use the newer types of cooking oil substitutes, so you can prepare the eggs without additional fat. These oil substitutes cut down both on the number of calories and on the saturated fat that butter or oil would usually provide. You can also prepare your eggs in a Teflon-coated nonstick frying pan.

CEREALS

Use any one of the following for one bread or cereal serving:

Ready-to-Eat Cereals

All Bran	½ cup	Puffed Rice	1 ½ cups
Bran Flakes	¾ cup	Puffed Wheat	1 ½ cups
Cheerios	1 cup	Raisin Bran	½ cup
Cornflakes	¾ cup	Rice Krispies	¾ cup
Grape Nut		Shredded	
Flakes	½ cup	Wheat	1 biscuit
Grape Nuts	¼ cup (1 ¼ bread serving)	Special K	1 cup
		Spoon-size	
Life	1 cup	Shredded Wheat	½ cup
Natural cereals	⅓ cup (without nuts)	Wheat Chex	½ cup (1 ½ bread serving)
Post Toasties	1 cup	Wheaties	¾ cup

Cooked Cereals

Cream of Wheat	½ cup	Oatmeal	½ cup
Farina	½ cup	Pettijohn's	½ cup
Grits	½ cup	Ralston	½ cup
Maltex	½ cup	Wheatena	½ cup
Malt-O-Meal	½ cup		

Note: The above amounts are for cereals after cooking.

This diet, as you can see by reading the meal plan, focuses on cereals and their equivalents, the variety of which is very large. Whether the cereals are protein enriched, vitamin fortified, dry, or cooked, they all provide good nutrition. Serving different types of cereal will add variety and interest to the meal.

Snacks can be largely cereal based. Certain starchy vegetables can be considered cereal equivalents; for example, beans, parsnips, peas, carrots, beets, onions, acorn squash, or winter squash. The large number of alternatives does require planning choices in order to stay within the diet and select an interesting cross-section of what is available. Since the list of cereals is so long, you can stay on the Natural Diet without ever eating oatmeal, or some other cereal that does not appeal to you.

SNACK FOODS

Any one of the following breads and cereal foods may be used as a snack for one serving of bread, provided your meal plan permits a snack.

> ½ bagel
> 2 Graham Crackers (2½-in. squares)
> 1 cup popcorn, popped (no added butter or margarine)
> 1 Dutch pretzel, or 6 3-ring, or 6 thin sticks
> 1 slice raisin bread, un-iced
> ½ cup ready-to-eat cereal (see cereal list)

Crackers

> 4 Melba Toast
> 6 round thins
> 3 Rye Krisps
> 10 Rye Thins
> 5 Saltines
> 3 soda crackers
> 12 Wheat Thins

MEATS

Choose from the following allowed meats (daily total 5 ounces meat, 6 ounces fowl or 7 ounces fish):

Beef
Crab, clams, lobster (occasionally)
Creamed cottage cheese
Egg whites, cholesterol-free eggs
Fish (if canned, drain oil)
Lamb
Lean ham

Low-fat cheeses
Oysters, scallops, shrimp
   (occasionally)
Pork
Poultry
Veal

Two ounces of skim-milk cottage cheese or low-fat cheese may be substituted for one ounce of the above meats.

Avoid the following meats and meat products, which are high in saturated fats:

All fatty meats
Bacon and sausage

Canned meat products
Commercially fried meats

Corned beef
Duck and goose
Egg yolk
Fish roe, including caviar
Fried fish or fowl
Full-fat cheese, including cream
   cheese
Luncheon meats, cold cuts, and
   hot dogs
Meats, canned or frozen, in gravy
   or sauce
Organ meats
Poultry skin
Spareribs

Since the amount of meat permitted is limited, be selective. It is best to choose lean, well-trimmed cuts of meat, either fresh or frozen. Meats can be baked, boiled, broiled, or roasted. Avoid fried meats or fried fish. Whatever fat is used in the preparation of the meat must be within the fat allowance. Generally speaking, fish contains fewer calories than beef, so fresh fish servings can be 50 percent larger than meat servings.

Take note of the list of meats and meat products which are high in saturated fats. Most of these are rich in calories as well and are best avoided. In special situations it is useful to limit quantities to whatever is appropriate to the occasion. For example, enjoy the shrimp at a cocktail party if you don't usually have them at home. Remember, a *long-range* diet means one that you can live with in reasonable comfort.

FRUITS

Use fresh, dried, cooked, canned, or frozen fruit to which neither sugar nor syrup has been added. (Usually a dried fruit serving is one-third to one-fourth the volume of the equivalent fresh fruit. A cooked fruit is equal to a fresh serving if no sugar or syrup has been added.) Read labels carefully. Use fruit or juice labeled "Unsweetened." Do not add sugar, honey, or syrup to fresh fruit.

The following equal one serving:

Apple	1 small (2-in. diameter)
Apple juice or cider	⅓ cup
Applesauce	½ cup
Apricots	4 halves
Banana	½ small
Berries	1 cup blackberries, ½ cup blueberries, ¾ cup raspberries, 1 cup strawberries
Cherries, fresh or canned	10 large or 15 small
Dates	2
Figs, canned	3 medium
Figs, dried	1 small
Grapefruit, fresh	½ small
Grapefruit sections, unsweetened	½ cup

Grapefruit juice	½ cup
Grape juice	¼ cup
Grapes	12 large or 20 small
Melons	¼ cantaloupe, ⅛ honeydew, 1 cup diced watermelon
Nectarine	1 medium
Orange, fresh	1 medium
Orange juice	½ cup
Peach	1 medium
Pear	2 halves
Pineapple	2 rings or ⅓ cup chunks
Plums	2 medium
Prune juice	¼ cup
Prunes, dried	2
Strawberries	1 cup
Raisins	2 Tbs.

Fruits are a welcome addition to any diet. Fresh fruits are preferable to canned fruits and are usually available all year round in most parts of the country. Be certain that prepared fruit is not packaged in syrup or sugar. It is not necessary to add sugar, honey, or syrup to fresh fruits—indeed, you may be pleasantly surprised to find how tasty the fruit is when it is properly and attractively served. Remember that fruits are extremely variable in their caloric content. For example, a cup of strawberries, which is high in water content, is the equivalent of only two tablespoons of raisins. Look again at the fruit serving list and adjust the quantity you eat to the equivalent of one serving. With a little interest and practice, you will soon be an expert at judging the relative caloric content of fruits. It does require rechecking the fruit list whenever you have a doubt.

BREADS AND CEREALS

Any one of the following foods equals one bread or cereal serving.

Bread, Starch, or Cereals

Biscuit (2-in. diameter)	1
Bread: enriched white, wheat, rye, pumpernickel, Italian, uniced raisin	1 slice
Cereal, cooked	½ cup
Cereal, puff-type, dry	¾ cup
Crackers: graham, 2½-in. square; saltines, 2-in. square	2 or 5 (see snack food list)
English muffin	½
Flour, cornmeal, dry grated bread crumbs	3 Tbs.

Grits, cooked	½ cup
Hamburger or hot dog roll	½
Hard roll	1 small or ½ large
Muffin (3-in. diameter)	1
Plain pancakes (4-in. diameter)	2
Plain waffle (7-in. diameter)	½
Popcorn, popped	1 cup
Rice, cooked	½ cup
Spaghetti, noodles, macaroni, cooked	½ cup

Make pancakes or waffles with allowed fats and oils. Omit one serving from fats and oils.

Starchy Vegetables

Baked beans (no pork or molasses)	¼ cup
Corn, small 4-in. ear	⅓ cup
Corn, whole kernel	⅓ cup
Dried beans and peas, cooked	½ cup
Lima beans	½ cup
Mixed vegetables	⅔ cup
Parsnips	⅔ cup

Bread, Cereal, or Starch

Potatoes, sweet	¼ cup
Potatoes, white, 2-in. diameter	1 small
Potatoes, white, mashed	½ cup

VEGETABLES

The following vegetables are low in calories and contain negligible amounts of carbohydrate, protein, or fat. Therefore, they may be eaten freely, that is, in normal amounts at mealtime or in between meals if desired. Margarine for seasoning vegetables must be within the fat allowed at the meal. Butter and salt may be used sparingly instead of margarine.

Artichokes	Chinese cabbage
Asparagus	Collard greens
Bean sprouts	Cucumbers
Beet greens	Dandelion greens
Broccoli	Eggplant
Brussels sprouts	Endive
Cabbage	Escarole
Cauliflower	Fennel
Celery	Kale
Chicory	Kohlrabi

Lettuce	Scallions
Mushrooms	Spinach
Mustard greens	Squash: summer, crookneck, flat
Okra	scalloped, straightneck, zucchini
Onions, green	String beans: green or yellow
Pepper, green	Swiss chard
Pickles, sour	Tomatoes, tomato juice, tomato
Radishes	puree
Romaine	Turnip greens
Sauerkraut	

The following vegetables contain some carbohydrate. They should be eaten in half-cup portions, and should be substituted for half a bread or starch serving.

Beets	Peas
Carrots	Winter squash (acorn)
Onions	

The vegetables on these lists can be eaten raw in almost any quantity. Usually one cup of cooked vegetables equals a serving. Almost unlimited, attractive, and nutritious, vegetables should not be overlooked. Some of the fat serving (margarine) can be used to decorate the vegetables. Vegetables provide bulk in the diet, a very important consideration for the sense of satiety. Because they contain vegetable fibers and are a natural source of vitamins and minerals as well as the roughage so important for good digestion, they are an important element in good nutrition. The variety of fresh, frozen, canned, and preserved vegetables is simply staggering. Their low cost and easy adaptation to any form of ethnic meal planning makes vegetables an important part of every dieter's meal planning.

BEVERAGES

Every adult should plan on having some low-fat milk daily. The diet calls for approximately two cups, but this can be modified to suit individual preferences. Milk is an excellent source of protein and can also supply calcium and vitamins. Some people are unable to tolerate milk; for them, skim milk yogurt, and cottage cheese are satisfactory alternatives. Milk makes good sense on a diet.

Drink any of the large variety of no-calorie beverages such as tea, coffee, or decaffeinated coffee (without cream and sugar, of course). Many recently introduced beverages have modified amounts of sugar and can be used occasionally. Read the labels. Water is important; your own thirst is a good guide to how much you should drink.

There is another kind of drinking for which your own thirst is not a good guide. I refer, of course, to alcoholic beverages. Some dieters assume that they can never drink on a diet. Before too long a sense of self-denial has doomed their fledgling dietary efforts. Relax—an occasional drink is not the end of the world or of a balanced, low-calorie diet.

Alcoholic beverages are derived mainly from cereal grains. Wine is the one exception, yet grapes can be considered part of the fruit allotment. There is no reason to deny yourself an occasional drink within the limits of your exchange pattern. For example, an ounce of Scotch or bourbon can be considered a cereal equivalent. Three ounces of wine would be a fruit equivalent. Try an ounce of brandy or cognac as an evening snack.

What is important is whether the drink has meaning to you. If one drink a day is an established pattern of behavior, then you need not deny yourself on the Natural Diet.

While it makes no sense to be a martyr over an occasional drink, the Natural Diet is not an open invitation to unlimited drinking. If you replace all your cereal intake with alcohol, then your liquid diet will be nutritionally inadequate. "All things in moderation, and moderation in all things" makes sense as far as your alcoholic and caloric intake are concerned.

FREE FOODS

The following can be used freely in addition to the foods on your meal plan.

Bouillon	Gelatin, unflavored
Carbonated beverages without sugar	Herbs
Carbonated or soda water	Mint
Chewing gum, sugarless	Mustard
Coffee (black)	Soy sauce
Flavorings	Spices

SAMPLE MENUS

In order to give you an idea of how the diet can be planned, following are seven sample daily menus to show you what can be done. It must be emphasized that these are not rigid menus but merely samples to give you an idea of how to go about following the diet. Part of the value of menu planning is nutritional insight. The best way to learn is to get your feet wet by planning your own menus. Whatever errors you may make are less important than your willingness to correct those errors, once you realize that your diet has not gone exactly as you planned.

Day 1

Breakfast

> ½ cup orange juice
> 1 ½ cups cornflakes
> 1 cup skim milk
> Coffee or tea

Lunch

> ½ cup cottage cheese
> 1 rye bagel, toasted
> Tossed salad with 1 Tbs. oil and vinegar
> 1 tsp. margarine
> 1 fresh orange
> Coffee, tea, or sugar-free soft drink

Dinner

> 3 oz. roast beef
> ½ cup rice with mushrooms, pimento, and green pepper
> 1 cup French-cut green beans
> Crispy cole slaw (use vinegar or lemon juice and artificial sweetener)
> 1 small dinner roll
> 1 tsp. margarine
> ⅓ cup unsweetened pineapple
> Coffee or tea

Snack

> 1 cup skim milk
> 1 cup popcorn

Day 2

Breakfast

> ½ grapefruit
> 1 cup oatmeal
> 1 cup skim milk
> Coffee or tea

Lunch

> 2 oz. roast turkey
> 2 slices whole wheat bread
> Leaf lettuce
> 2 tsp. mayonnaise
> Dill pickle spears
> 1 small apple
> Coffee, tea, or sugar-free soft drink

Dinner

> Tomato bouillon
> 3 oz. baked pork chop
> ½ cup baked sweet potato
> Broccoli spears
> 1 tsp. margarine
> ½ cup frozen blueberries
> Coffee or tea

Snack

> 1 cup skim milk
> 2 graham crackers

Day 3

Breakfast

- ½ banana
- 2 cups Life cereal
- 1 cup skim milk
- Coffee or tea

Lunch

- 2 oz. cold roast beef
- 1 onion bun
- Mustard
- 1 tsp. margarine
- Sliced tomatoes and lettuce
- 1 Tbs. French dressing
- 12 tokay grapes
- Coffee, tea, or sugar-free soft drink

Dinner

- 4 oz. roast chicken
- Succotash: ½ cup lima beans and ⅓ cup cut corn
- Tossed salad
- 1 Tbs. Italian dressing
- ½ cup unsweetened applesauce
- Coffee or tea

Snack

- 1 cup skim milk
- 12 Wheat Thins crackers

Day 4

Breakfast

- ½ cup orange juice
- 1 cup bran flakes
- 1 cup skim milk
- Coffee or tea

Lunch

- ½ cup tuna fish with chopped celery, onion, dill pickle
- 2 tsp. mayonnaise
- 10 Saltines
- 1 tangerine
- Coffee, tea, or sugar-free soft drink

Dinner

- 3 oz. veal scallopini (veal steak, tomatoes, mushrooms, green pepper)
- ½ cup wild and long-grain rice
- 1 small dinner roll
- 1 cup leaf spinach
- 1 tsp. margarine
- 2 unsweetened peach halves
- Coffee or tea

Snack

- 1 cup skim milk
- ½ bagel

Day 5

Breakfast
¼ cup prune juice
2 Shredded Wheat biscuits
1 cup skim milk
Coffee or tea

Lunch
½ cup cottage cheese
Lettuce wedge
1 Tbs. French dressing
2 slices raisin bread
1 tsp. margarine
⅓ cup unsweetened pineapple
Coffee, tea, or sugar-free soft
    drink

Dinner
3 oz. baked ham
2 small parslied potatoes
1 cup French-cut green beans
Sauerkraut salad
1 tsp. margarine
½ cup unsweetened mandarin
    oranges
Coffee or tea

Snack
1 cup skim milk
6 3-ring pretzels

Day 6

Breakfast
½ cup grapefruit
1 cup Ralston
1 cup skim milk
Coffee or tea

Lunch
½ cup cholesterol-free scram-
    bled egg
2 slices whole wheat bread
2 tsp. margarine
Sliced tomato, cucumber, and
    onion salad
Fresh pear
Coffee, tea, or sugar-free soft
    drink

Dinner
3 oz. meatballs (ground sirloin)
½ cup spaghetti in tomato
    sauce
1 slice garlic bread
Steamed zucchini squash and
    Italian onion
1 tsp. margarine
¾ cup frozen, unsweetened
    melon balls
Coffee or tea

Snack
1 cup skim milk
1 cup popcorn

Day 7

Breakfast

   ½ banana
   2 cups Special K cereal
   1 cup skim milk
   Coffee or tea

Lunch

   2 oz. lean ham
   1 onion roll
   Mustard
   2 tsp. mayonnaise
   Lettuce, dill pickle chips
   Fresh orange
   Coffee, tea, or sugar-free soft drink

Dinner

   3 oz. broiled steak
   1 small baked potato
   1 cup asparagus cuts and tips
   Crispy slaw
   1 small hard roll
   1 tsp. margarine
   1 cup frozen strawberries
   Coffee or tea

Snack

   1 cup buttermilk
   20 Rye Thins

PUTTING THE NATURAL DIET TO WORK

Your first decision has to be that you *will* have breakfast, preferably with your family. You may feel that there are never enough hours in a day. Skipping breakfast or eating a doughnut and gulping down a cup of coffee while standing is common behavior that, however, results in more calories and less balanced nutrition. *Plan on starting the day by sitting down to breakfast.*

This simple first step may require some preparation and behavior modification in order to accomplish the important objective of bringing the family together as a unit. Dieters need support and input from those around them, and breakfast is a prime time to accomplish this. To do so, everyone will have to make some compromises and adjustments: The dieter must wake up early enough so that he or she can eat before going to work. Your children must be disciplined enough (by themselves hopefully, but by parents' insistence if necessary) to arrive at the table at about the same time, dressed and ready for school. The meal preparer should sit down and eat with the family instead of serving as hired help. This may require modification of the morning menu, but cereals, cooked or dry, lend themselves to easy preparation. The table can be set the evening before to save time—convince the children.

Almost everyone will lose weight on the 1250 calories the diet provides. As the dieter approaches ideal weight, larger portions of cereals and fruit can be added. For example, adding a cereal equivalent and a fruit equivalent to each meal and the evening snack, will add about 500 to 600 calories and bring the daily allowance close to a maintenance level for most adults (1800 calories).

If the problem is too little weight loss, the reduction of two cereal and one fruit serving a day will bring the intake close to 1,000 calories, low enough for almost anyone to lose weight steadily and satisfactorily.

These deviations will *not* result in inadequate nutrition and they will *not* result in an increased intake of cholesterol.

BREAKFAST

Breakfast consists of cereal, usually one or two ounces per person, juice, and beverage (see meal plan). Modifications to suit various family members are quite simple; the children will get more milk and larger cereal and fruit servings. If you are short, (five feet or so) and weigh about fifty-five kilograms (121 pounds), stick to a low range of intake; four ounces of skim milk, one ounce of cereal, four ounces of juice, and a noncaloric beverage will suffice. Taller (five feet seven inches or more) or heavier people (above 150 pounds) can have two ounces of the cereal, eight ounces of skim milk, and a larger portion of juice. Some adjustments for your activity, sex, life-style, and initial weight all make sense.

Low-cholesterol egg substitutes for the cereal portion of breakfast provide additional variety. They are rich in protein and have moderate amounts of fat. Different brands vary quite a bit, some containing about 100 calories per egg equivalent, while others are advertised as having only thirty-five calories. A good deal of this seemingly large difference is explained when one examines the nutritional data listed on the box. It is apparent that the manufacturers of the lower-calorie product assign a smaller weight to their egg equivalent. This also means there is less to eat per serving, and so the differences are magnified by the variations in the definition of what is an egg.

Certainly breakfast need not be monotonous. Ideally, breakfast should provide approximately ten grams of protein, which, on the Natural Diet, you will get from the cereal and the skim or low-fat milk allowed in the meal plan. Studies have demonstrated that adequate nutrition helps avoid the doldrums which often afflict the dieter who literally starves until the dinner hour, and then spends the rest of the evening gorging.

LUNCH

Lunch is an important meal which is often skipped or purposely neglected by the dieter. For many housewives, lunch consists of a series of snacks and nibbles, beginning with mid-morning coffee and pastry and ending with a continuous tasting of whatever is cooking for supper. This "cycle of nibbles" is a common problem. Behavior modification is called for here—you must sit down and eat lunch *once*.

It is important to plan on a lunch which will provide you with good nutrition and yet be low in calories. Lunch can be varied. The menu includes two ounces of meat, two ounces of cereal, a fruit serving, a vegetable serving, a fat serving, and a no-calorie beverage. Pick from the alternatives within each group. Two ounces of meat and two slices of bread can become a meat, fish, or fowl sandwich. The lettuce and tomatoes of a vegetable serving can be added to a sandwich or tossed in a salad. The salad can be embellished with a low-calorie dressing, or simple vinegar or lemon juice. Fruit makes a pleasant, low-calorie dessert.

Cereals such as rice, spaghetti, or bagels accommodate a variety of meals such as a Chinese meal with fruit and vegetable, an Italian meal with stewed tomatoes, or a toasted bagel with smoked salmon. All provide a satisfying, nutritional lunch.

As you can see, eating nutritiously balanced meals does not necessitate rigid adherence to a fixed menu. Indeed, the Natural Diet's variety and your imagination make the diet an adventure rather than a burden. When you accept the diet for life, you can use your energies creatively.

Lunch is an important meal for many reasons. It provides a break in your day, no matter what your job or home responsibilities are. Regular meals do not mean more food intake; often they are lower in calories than nighttime nibbles.

DINNER

Dinner is usually the most critical meal of a diet. It represents the largest meal of the day and requires the most planning and preparation. (This is not true in some other cultures, where the midday meal is the largest, as in Greece and Italy, for example.) Individuals who are content eating the same breakfast for years are often careful to plan varied late-evening meals. Similarly, the evening meal has special significance for some families. It is often the only meal that the entire family shares in, reviewing the day's activities and exchanging experiences. It can be a pleasant introduction to a relaxed evening at home, or a continuation of the armed-truce tension in a troubled household. Your spouse, children, parents, and friends can either help you with your diet or torpedo your effort, and dinner is where it happens.

Evening mealtime is often the make-or-break time for the dieter. All too often it serves merely as the prelude to continuous nibbling for the entire evening. This is especially true of the obese person who feels virtuous as a result of fasting all day. It is this destructive, self-defeating nighttime eating that the Natural Diet can help you overcome, because once you have established a pattern of having healthful, satisfying meals for breakfast, lunch, and dinner, you will not feel that nagging hunger that causes you to add to your calorie intake by that constant nibbling.

Dinner will require your most conscientious effort. You can see from the meal plan that dinner contains three ounces of meat, four onces of fowl, or five ounces of fish. Plan on eating less than twenty ounces of meat a week, and you'll soon be saving money as well as losing weight. The fowl, either chicken or turkey, should not include the skin. Almost any variety of fish, fresh or frozen, is permissible. You'll note that there are two cereal servings for the dinner meal, which can include rice, bread, pasta, squash, or potato. The vegetable serving can be increased to satisfy your hunger. Never hesitate to take a second helping of asparagus, broccoli, Brussels sprouts, eggplant, mushrooms, or spinach. The extra calories are minimal and you will not have a sense of deprivation. Plan on having fruit for dessert (you *can* eat dessert), or try one of the dessert recipes in the back of the book. You really will not be hungry when you leave the table. If after dinner you still have late-night cravings, you are allowed one snack. You'll be off to bed without feeling like a martyr, but you will not have the insomnia of hunger either. The midnight "hungries" (remember Dagwood Bumstead and his sandwiches?) won't yank you out of bed. When you are done for the day you will have eaten 1,250 calories, consumed adequate protein and vitamins, and lost some weight. It will be slow but steady and you won't have to worry about being under-nourished.

Going out for dinner or entertaining at home are special circumstances. Every dieter has been to a party and said no to very attractively served food while everyone else was eating voraciously. With the Natural Diet, this is really not necessary. If you are adhering to your meal plan conscientiously, deviations for a special occasion will not be significant in the long run. Stick to some of the less rich hors d'oeuvres and try to limit the amount you have.

If you really feel that you will be deprived by sticking to your diet when you are being entertained, then go ahead and enjoy the party and just redouble your efforts thereafter. When you know that you are going to a party next weekend, you might plan on denying yourself a few of your snacks during the preceding two days. An important aspect of this diet is not to walk around like a P.O.W., as if you were missing all the good things in life. Since the diet is a long-range one, short-term interruptions are less meaningful. However, if you convince yourself that ten dietary indiscretions a week are normal for you, then you probably haven't decided to go on a diet.

Anyone who assumes that a diet will quickly and painlessly lop off fifty pounds of unwanted fat is unrealistic and doomed to disappointment. The most successful diets are like good interpersonal relationships: they wear well over a long period of time and are truly something you can live with. Fad diets are like brief affairs: they do not last because they don't fulfill your needs.

3.

Keeping a Diet Diary

When at the table we never repent for having eaten or drunk too little.
—Thomas Jefferson

An important adjunct to the Natural Diet is keeping an accurate diet diary. A diet diary is a record of what you eat. Because you will soon forget what you ate for dinner (or what you ate between lunch and dinner) the day before yesterday, you must keep a *daily* diet diary.

Most dieters are absolutely astonished at the helpfulness of the diary. As you write down what you eat, you become aware of your eating patterns. The most difficult step is overcoming inertia; thereafter, the effort of keeping a diary is modest. Many dieters are reluctant to spend time writing down what they eat; they are less reluctant to spend time preparing and eating snacks. As a matter of fact, dieters think about food more often than their slim counterparts. The diary is a record of what you are already doing. It is easy, manageable, and necessary.

A simple sheet of 8½×11 paper will do, or you can use 3×5 index cards, or design your own sheets (a sheet we have used successfully in our dietary research is included in this chapter). Every time you eat or drink, you must write it down. Note the time you eat, the place you eat, and your physical position—standing, sitting, or lying. Write down whether you are eating alone or with someone else. Note your mood—were you angry, bored, tired, depressed, or happy? Were you starving or were you eating out of habit? Were you snacking for want of something better to do? Describe the food and specify the portion size. If you don't weigh your portions, you can guess, using cups, ounces, or inches.

Record what, when, how much, with whom, and why you eat: "I was hungry," "It was lunchtime," "I was bored." Then describe how you felt afterwards. For example: "I loved it," "It wasn't worth the calories," "I'm still bored." It should be brief and to the point.

Such a record discourages thoughtless eating. Research studies done at the University of Pennsylvania Behavioral Weight Control Clinic have shown that most people lose weight when they keep diet diaries.

All overweight people wish for miracles; new fad diets always make promises, but there is usually very little data to support these extravagant claims. These diets cure obesity about as well as vitamins cure cancer.

Everyone has heard the standard cry of the fat person: "I don't understand why I gain weight, I eat no more than everyone else. I eat like a bird." Most people who eat like sparrows eventually resemble sparrows. If you don't eat, you can't gain weight. How can you be sure what you don't eat? You can be sure only by writing down everything that you do eat!

Recording what you eat changes your behavior. The diet diary forces you to focus on what you eat, when you eat, and why you eat. Keeping a diet diary will identify patterns of overeating and help you concentrate on changing undesirable patterns. If you discover that you eat while watching TV, you can focus on changing that pattern. A diet diary is your personal eating inventory.

Don't lie to yourself. The diet diary is not designed for self-incrimination. It is designed to help you understand when you are eating, what you are eating, and why you are eating. If possible, you should share this information with a doctor, a nutritionist, or a co-dieter. If you feel that you do not wish to share this information, you can review it yourself several days later. It's a good trick to keep a diary for a time, put it aside, and analyze it critically a week or two later. Some people are shocked to learn that they have actually had almost fifty different meals or snacks within a week. If you are honest with yourself, you will certainly learn something about your own eating habits.

Once you are aware of your eating habits, moods, and behavior, modifications are easier. Remember, it is the long haul that matters. Try to be patient. There is no need to make unrealistic demands on yourself, but there are reasons to modify your behavior if it causes overweight. For example, always shop with a full stomach, buy fewer rich snacks, and leave the junk food on the supermarket shelves. At home, store those rich snack foods that you do buy behind fruits and vegetables. In an experiment at the University of Pennsylvania, high-calorie desserts were first placed in front of the low-calorie desserts. Most people chose high-calorie desserts. After several days, the cafeteria reversed the placement so that the low-calorie desserts were at the front of the counter and the high-calorie desserts hidden at the back. During the next several days, more people chose low-calorie desserts. Obviously, convenience has something to do with the foods we choose. This kind of behavior modification is almost painless.

The diet diary can be an asset in balancing your weekend excesses. If you know that your calorie intake will be 1,250 calories a day, you have a point of departure. If you plan a party Saturday night or a large family dinner on Sunday, you can make some minor adjustments in the snacks during the five weekdays. Plan your diet ahead of time. This is not to say that all the calories should be transferred lock, stock, and barrel into one or two sessions on the weekend. It does mean, however, that with some planning you can have your diet and party as well. You can arrange your meals so that you eat mostly low-calorie foods on the days before your party or large dinner. If you are strict and don't allow yourself to slip back into your old patterns during those days, a few extra calories on the weekend, if they cannot be avoided, will not be all that detrimental to your diet. But do not exceed a week's calories in a week. Starvation is not necessary; good planning is.

Additionally, a diet diary encourages you to personalize your portions. If you are five foot four inches and your husband is six foot two, there is a significant difference in the number of calories that you each require. People's activities vary and you must build into your diet portions that are appropriate to your activities. If you want a piece of apple pie and know that one piece contains 300 calories, you have a decision to make. You might be able to tolerate half a piece—150 calories—without too much damage to your diet plan, and your larger, more active husband might better tolerate the 450 calories of one and a half pieces.

The diary helps you learn when to leave food on your plate. If you are served a great big Idaho potato, and you really know that a medium sized potato is your caloric serving, then you know you should leave half the potato on your plate. You can learn many caloric equivalents as you continue to diet. (Check as often as necessary the Food Composition table in the Appendix, which lists caloric values for most foods.) A small piece of chocolate candy will cost about 100 calories; so will thirty spears of asparagus. Obviously, if you are looking for a balanced and satisfying meal, the asparagus is a better choice. Sometimes, however, the little piece of chocolate is more meaningful. The important thing is not to have both. Have the one you really want for whatever reason, but learn to make a decision. With a little effort you will be able to incorporate your preferences into your diet.

Tables of 100 grams or 3 ½ ounces of foods are very useful. With practice, you will soon find that a small Manhattan cocktail equals a glass of orange juice or a large potato. You will also find that you can eat considerably larger portions of vegetables without losing control of your diet.

You will lose weight and keep it off. Long-term maintenance is really what

SAMPLE DIET DIARY PAGE

Date	Time	Meal	Where	Physical Position	With Whom	Food Description	Quantity	Mood

you want. Using a diet diary in conjunction with the Natural Diet will enable you to reach the weight you've always fantasized about but have never been able to maintain.

The shape your body is in is too important to be treated in a cavalier fashion. Since you are what you eat, now is the time to learn when to stop eating.

4.

Calories Do Count

More die from the pot than from poverty.

—Babylonian Talmud

Every dieter must understand that a calorie is a calorie is a calorie. Calories *do* count. Successful dieting requires as much knowledge as willpower, but you must first *want* to lose weight. Your motivation is most important.

Many overweight people believe that they eat very little, but when they say this they are referring primarily to volume, not caloric value. There is a 4,000 percent difference in the number of calories per gram between very, very low-calorie and high-calorie foods. For example, lettuce has less than twenty calories per four-ounce serving, and butter has more than 800 calories per four-ounce serving. Clearly, four ounces is more butter than you would serve, but the differences do count. Two pats of butter, which is an average serving, contain 100 calories. A twenty-calorie serving of butter would hardly be visible, while 100 calories of lettuce would weigh about a pound and fill a very large salad bowl.

The only way to lose weight and to maintain a desirable new weight is to change your eating habits. Fasting works only during the fasts. Many drastic diets accomplish only water losses. Once you start eating the way you did before, you'll soon weigh what you did before.

Habits, especially food habits, are difficult to break, and all of us have certain personal preferences. It is not necessary to eliminate all the foods you like. It *is* necessary to reduce sharply the amount of meat, especially beef and pork, that you eat. In order to achieve the goals of this diet, you must substitute fish and fowl for much of the meat you used to eat. Ethnic preferences can easily be accommodated; one serving of cereal can be any of the following: half a bagel, a half cup of cooked spaghetti, a half cup of grits, or a half cup of rice. You may choose any of these, and in fact you should try them all—at different meals. Eating foods that are both interesting and tasteful avoids monotony; anyone will get tired of having just steak and salad meal after meal. Variety permits you to stick to the diet.

By reducing the amount of meat to about five ounces a day, several important gains are achieved, one of which is a reduction in total calories. Every food contains calories. The energy potential of calories is stored as fat when caloric intake exceeds that which can be metabolized. Meat, despite what you have believed up to this point, is very rich. It is high in protein, fat, and calories. It is easy to eat many meat calories without realizing it, because meat calories come in a rather concentrated form. Everyone who has enjoyed a steak in a fine restaurant realizes that large portions can be finished in the course of a pleasant meal. The steaks that you eat probably average between twelve and fifteen ounces and represent well over 1,000 calories. It is less likely that anyone is going to sit down and eat a quart of oatmeal, a whole box of cornflakes, or eight servings of rice in a single meal—which is the amount you would need to eat to get the same number of calories. In addition, cereal supplies the body with minerals and vitamins that you cannot get from meat. This is a very important consideration. And you can easily get protein from other foods.

The protein in fish and fowl is of exactly the same quality as the protein in meat; you do not have to eat meat in order to get adequate protein. Complete protein is also present in milk and milk products, as well as in eggs.

We all know that protein is necessary in a healthy diet, but we have been conditioned to believe that the only way to get protein is to eat vast quantities of meat. This is simply not the case. Protein is made up of thirty-two amino acids, all but eight of which are manufactured by the human body. These remaining eight amino acids we must get from the food we eat. Many foods that we normally do not think of as containing protein do, indeed, contain *some* of these eight amino acids—they are not considered complete because they do not have all eight. However, when these foods are combined with certain other foods that have the missing amino acids (but that also do not contain complete protein), *voilà*—the combination becomes a complete protein.

The proteins in grains and in certain nuts and seeds also complement each other. The protein in dairy products combines very efficiently with that in cereal grains, bringing the total protein content up to more than what you would get if you ate each food separately. An important thing to remember, however, is that in order to obtain this complementary benefit, the foods you are combining must be eaten together, at the same meal.

Now, I'm not suggesting that everyone become a vegetarian (though this is some of the theory behind what makes it possible to be a healthy vegetarian). This discussion should show you, however, that it is quite possible to lower your intake of meat and raise your level of health. If you are going to modify your eating behavior, education about good nutrition will be a big help.

No diet can possibly be complete without three things: first, motivation; second, a specific, nutritionally correct diet; third, and equally important, reinforcement that comes from continued meetings with either a physician, a nutritionist, or other members of a group who are dealing with the same problem. In a group, people support and reinforce each other through the difficult phases. This is very important because it is not unusual for people to plateau—level off—at some point even though they are religiously adhering to a diet. It is amazing how often intelligent people make unintentional errors which can frustrate weight loss.

Patience is an absolute necessity during the early phases of a diet. If you are convinced that you are following the diet and are not losing weight, do not despair. There are many explanations for this, including the fact you may be eating more calories than you think (a diet diary will be useful in this case).

You must be realistic in your diet goals. Some simple mathematical considerations are appropriate here. An average sedentary male of 154 pounds (seventy kilograms) will require approximately 2,400 calories per day to maintain his body weight. He would use more if he was very young and less if he was older, but 2,400 calories is a good approximation. An average woman (five foot four inches) who weighs 120 pounds (fifty-five kilograms) will naturally require significantly fewer calories. Many women shorter than five feet will not lose weight unless their calorie intake is below 1,400 calories a day. If the woman were only five feet tall and burned 1,500 calories a day she would have a daily deficit of only 100 calories on a 1,400 calorie diet. This means that she would require thirty-five days on a 1,400 calorie diet to lose one pound. If she had an indiscretion or two it would take longer. Short people are at a real disadvantage in terms of their ability to lose weight. Assuming that the five-foot-four woman in question burns 1,850 calories and consumes 1,500, she would then eliminate 350 calories a day. A man with an intake of 1,700 calories would enjoy a 700-calorie deficit a day (2,400−1,700=700). This difference is due to physical size and activity.

Because 3,500 calories equals approximately one pound of body weight, it is easy to see how a man and a woman on the same diet would react differently. Unfortunately, the woman would lose weight only half as fast as the man, although she ate less. Since it would take ten days for her to have a cumulative deficit of 3,500 calories, she would lose approximately three pounds a month on such a diet. Clearly 1,500 calories is a significant intake and if it were reduced to 1,150, she would then lose weight at the rate of one to two pounds a week, which is about the same weight loss that the man would accomplish.

There are certain other considerations, such as the loss of water weight. This may be delayed for a relatively long time and is not always observable during the initial phases of dieting.

Once the simple mathematics of weight reduction are understood, it then becomes apparent that anything which helps burn more calories (like exercise) can improve the results of dieting significantly. Walking a mile burns approximately 100 calories; walking rapidly burns somewhat more. Assuming that someone is able to burn 100 additional calories a day, in a month a deficit of 3,500 calories would be accumulated. Done every day, the same pattern would result in a loss of twelve pounds a year with no change in diet. Exercise, contrary to popular belief, does not increase appetite. If you exercise regularly, you may eat less, not more.

Activities such as bowling, which require little substantial effort, are not significant exercise. The contribution of the effort expended is small and most of the time is spent waiting passively. Exercise alone will accomplish only minimal and painfully slow weight loss. It is possible, however, by planning on walking whenever possible, climbing stairs in the building in which you work or live, and using some of your recreational time for endurance-type exercise (swimming or walking), to accelerate your weight loss.

A recent study examined the roles of exercise and diet individually and in combination. The authors (W.B. Zuti and L.A. Goldring, "Comparing Diet and Exercise as Weight Reduction Tools," in *The Physician and Sports Medicine*, 1976, pp. 49-53, published by Kansas and Kent State Universities) gathered twenty-five volunteers, women between the ages of twenty-five and forty-two who were twenty to forty pounds overweight. They carefully calculated the number of calories each woman actually required to maintain her weight. They divided the women into three approximately equal groups. Each woman in the exercise group ate no less than usual but exercised enough to burn up a total of 500 calories a day. The diet group reduced their daily caloric intake by 500 calories. Finally, in the combination group, 250 calories a day were burned by exercise and the dietary intake was decreased by 250 calories.

All three groups were followed for sixteen weeks. The final results showed that each group lost the same amount of weight, averaging about twelve pounds.

This demonstrates that some weight loss can be accomplished by diet and some by exercise. Notice the combined effect, and that the weight loss approximates what would be expected mathematically. The loss is slow, steady, and within a predictable range.

5.

Alternative Eating Patterns

Man can live without spices, but not without wheat.
—Midrash: Psalms 2:16

Explore your motives for dieting. Do you diet for good health? Because your friends are thin? Because you'll be beautiful when you are thin? Each of these motives is valid; often several motives contribute to the decision to diet.

It may surprise you to know that not everybody wants to be thin. Many obese people are afraid to become thin. For them obesity has become a protection from anxiety. Some use obesity to avoid sex, to avoid military service, or to manipulate members of their families.

PSYCHOLOGICAL FACTORS

SELF-IMAGE

Some obese people simply have decided that they are not fat. True, some overweight people are not fat; their incremental weight is largely muscle mass. But most people's weight problems have little to do with muscles. If you take off all your clothes and stand in front of a full-length mirror, you can see how fat you are. We all give ourselves the benefit of the doubt, assuming we are really muscular when we are, in reality, fat. How often have you heard a fat person describe himself as "big boned"? It's time to stop kidding yourself. Big bones and large muscles aside, fat is fat. Many fat people decide that obesity is a temporary problem that will magically go away. They seek a miracle drug or await a miracle diet. There is no magic. The fat is real; the painless or quick cure is fantasy.

Preoccupation with food, and eating food, is always a problem. Most people who are overweight deny that they eat as much as they do. Keep an accurate diet diary! Many fat people weigh themselves several times a day; others avoid the scale altogether. Checking your weight regularly must also become part of your new approach to dieting.

EATING PATTERNS

Obesity follows a pattern that begins in childhood. We associate size with maturity, so children are pressured to eat, often to excess. This overfeeding encourages the development of large numbers of fat cells, which remain throughout adult life. Many children's stories encourage food fantasies. Remember Hansel and Gretel? As children we learn that food is good—and more food is better. As adults we must learn to eat for nutrition, not for psychotherapy. Gratification need not be rich in calories.

In childhood, food is a source of reassurance, comfort, reward, and love. Withdraw food and you withdraw love. Adult life is much more complex. Food and love are no longer synonomous, but some of us continue to think of food as a reward. We must develop satisfactory alternatives to food as our major source of gratification. Maturity means developing appropriate responses to stress and frustrations, developing means other than eating of reducing anxiety. Modifying eating behavior really means finding a better way of dealing with life.

Most obese people do not have to be hungry to eat. For them, food takes on a value of its own. They often measure the success of a party or a wedding by the quality and quantity of food served.

Half the population of this country eats, drinks, and smokes excessively. People believe food gives strength and diet causes weakness. This is nonsense. Well-balanced, adequate diets only make you lose weight. You don't have to be undernourished.

FOOD AND EMOTIONS

Obese individuals are always planning to start a diet "tomorrow." They begin their day with willpower; by late afternoon they feel deprived and anxious. Unsuccessful dieters assume that they lack willpower. Actually, what they often lack is information for a long-range nutritional approach. Starting the day by starving merely intensifies the sense of deprivation dieters often feel.

As children have fairy-tale food fantasies, adults have literary and mythical ones. Not all of them are positive. In Greek mythology, Cronus ate his children in order to prevent them from competing with him. Statements in our vocabulary include "I can't swallow that" or "He bit off more than he could chew," all of which emphasize eating out of proportion to caloric and nutritional needs. Eating has become a national pastime as well as a linguistic idiom.

Successful dieting demands increased self-awareness and maturity. It means learning enough about what you eat and why you eat, so that you can make intelligent choices. The people around you—some well intentioned, some not—may sabotage your efforts. Your friends may tell you your face looks thinner, not your hips, or your husband may buy you a box of chocolates to celebrate your ten-pound weight loss after six weeks of dieting. As a person becomes thin, clothing, dress, and life-styles change, and so do interpersonal relationships. Not everyone around you can tolerate these changes. Many men find themselves threatened by a stylishly dressed, slender woman. Some women will be jealous of their skinny friends of either sex. Remember: changing your eating behavior *does* change your life and the lives of those who are close to you. You will have to learn to expect and reject the well-meaning friend or relative who encourages you to have "just one more helping." Hostesses often feel slighted if you eat with less gusto than they feel is appropriate after they "slaved over a hot stove." You can certainly expect comments, some complimentary and some snide, if you deign to pass up dessert! You must learn to tolerate and withstand attempts to get you to eat more than you know is good for you, whatever the motiviation of the people involved. In a recent study, volunteers who drank equal volumes of high- and low-calorie liquid formulas could not distinguish between the two. Their feelings of fullness or hunger were unrelated to caloric intake. In other words, additional calories do not necessarily make you feel less hungry or more full.

People who are highly responsive to the smell and taste of food are more likely to gain weight than less sensitive people. Many obese people have just this problem. They have a heightened responsiveness to food, and their interest in food is more easily aroused. If you are aware of this, you will avoid shopping when hungry, you will keep candy out of the home, and you will place especially favorite foods in an inconvenient location. Once you have identified your own problem, you can set about resolving it.

SOCIAL FACTORS

Societal patterns also influence weight. The incidence of obesity varies with sex (females more than males), with religious subdivisions (Lutherans tend to be more obese than Episcopalians), and with income (very poor more than very rich). Many more poor women are obese than rich women. One of the reasons—and there are many—is that peer pressure for having a slim figure is greater among affluent women. Wealthy women tend to be more clothes conscious, and expensive clothes are modeled by thin mannequins. Poor women tend to utilize cheaper foods, which are often higher in caloric content. Rich women have the time and money to engage in a variety of sports and exercises; they often join health clubs. Poor women are more often trapped at home and they often have less gratification and more frustration in their role as housewives.

Researchers have found that 40 percent of children with one obese parent are obese. If both parents are obese, then 80 percent of the children are obese. If both parents are of normal weight, only 7 percent of the children are obese. About 80 percent of these obese children will go on to become obese adults. While there is a heredity factor in obesity, habit is also important, as is your style of living. Weight can be controlled by diet and physical exercise. While you are influenced by genetics, you are not predestined to follow in your parents' footsteps. You can and should control your own weight.

Behavior modification, an excellent way to achieve permanent weight loss, is easier in a group setting. The group provides for social contacts and a way to blow off steam. The dieter can confess food-related guilts and neurotic feelings to fellow sufferers. It takes a fat person to really know the problems, not a cold, distant, holier-than-thou diet doctor. The group can influence the dieter as no parental figure or physician can. If the group is successful, it will result in flexibility in the approach to dieting that will avoid the feast-or-famine approach.

An important point to remember is that not everyone will have a perfect figure after dieting. Failure to understand this can lead to unnecessary unhappiness. Often a dieter will assume that the attainment of normal weight will bring instant popularity. At the same weight of 110 pounds, two five-foot-three young women may have entirely different physiques. One may be extremely well proportioned; another young woman with the same weight and height may have very heavy legs and be poorly proportioned. It is important to realize that attaining your ideal weight will not automatically bring you health, wealth, and happiness.

There is such a thing as going overboard, also. A young lady in her twenties had gained some weight in college and decided she was obese. She went on a starvation diet until she became emaciated. Despite all efforts to reassure her that she was not obese, she would force herself to vomit after eating in order to maintain her weight loss. Finally she required hospitalization to reverse this destructive process. She envisioned herself as obese even after she weighed eighty pounds. Of course, this woman had complex psychological problems.

Another problem the dieter must face is that of returning to previous eating patterns. Weight loss does not occur in a straight line; even on this Natural Diet, weight loss will be irregular and erratic. It is very discouraging to know that you have followed the diet for two weeks and have lost only half a pound or no weight at all. Feeling somehow doomed to failure despite your best efforts, you may very well go back to eating as you did before. If you resist, however, you will be rewarded with a successful weight loss rather than another failure.

Following the Natural Diet and keeping a diet diary are the stepping-stones to achieving the weight you want. This means changing your eating behavior, which many have done with gratifying results. For example, one thirty-nine-year-old female, who is five-foot-one, found that on the Natural Diet she began to think of herself as having a better body image and being healthy. She felt that the diet was eminently more satisfying and more workable than her previous attempts at dieting. She was able to maintain a diet diary without difficulty. During the diet, upon which she lost ten pounds, she felt much more vibrant and found that she could get along on the five ounces of meat beautifully. She especially enjoyed having the sandwich for lunch, since previous diets had specifically restricted her from any form of carbohydrates. Overall, she felt better and was able to function better.

6.
Eating Out and Other Adventures

Live in measure, and laugh at the mediciners.
Nothing contributes more to health than a temperate diet.

—James Kelly

Eating out should be, and usually is, a pleasure. However, many people wrongly believe that they cannot stay on a diet unless they never eat out, or unless they sit and drink black coffee while everyone else eats. Similarly, many modern dieters feel that starvation, self-denial, and a strictly limited list of permitted foods are the only way to lose weight. In reality, the more varied and flexible your diet, the more likely you are to stick with it. Don't concentrate on what you can't eat; instead, enjoy a large variety of permitted foods. The more you know about foods the more choices you will have.

Another self-defeating attitude is that the dieter must eat the same meals at home, day after day, because of the belief that only certain limited foods, prepared only in certain limited ways, are low enough in calories to fit into a diet plan. Such a belief, as you must be aware by now, goes completely contrary to all the tenets of the Natural Diet. You can eat exciting, varied foods, both at home and in restaurants, and stay on the diet, and lose weight.

Let's go to your favorite restaurant and go through the menu together: The first item is usually soup or an appetizer. You can have these if you follow a few basic rules. Stick to clear soups or the noncreamed, vegetable varieties. Ethnic varieties of vegetable soups such as minestrone, chicken soup with rice, or consommés are fine. Beet soup or borscht, tomato soups, or Manhattan clam chowder are acceptable alternatives. If you prefer an appetizer, you can substitute a fresh fruit cocktail, a shrimp cocktail, or smoked fish. Have a glass of dry white wine instead of a fruit equivalent today. One three-ounce wine serving can be considered a cereal or a fruit. Salads of every sort are available and can be topped with fresh lemon juice or oil and vinegar to taste. Low-calorie salad dressings may also be available. Vegetables and cereals are always available and add nutritious variety. Remember, for the purposes of this diet, hard rolls, French or Italian bread, old-fashioned rye, wheat crackers, pumpernickel, spaghetti, bagels, and grits are all cereals.

For lunch you can have any sandwich made with turkey, tuna fish, or lean roast beef. When you are dining out in the evening, the main course should be fresh broiled fish or meat or roast chicken. If the restaurant serves an excessively large steak, there are several realistic alternatives. I've found it pleasant and economical to split a main course with my wife. The average meat serving is about twelve ounces—enough for any two people. If you eat alone, just make up your mind to order the smallest portion you can. (A child's portion may injure your pride, but it makes sense in terms of cost and calories.) If there is no alternative to the full-size steak, then plan on eating half of it and taking the rest home in a doggie bag for the next day's meal. If you're reluctant to do that, it's wiser to leave half the meat in your plate than to store it as fat in your person. Skip the main dishes that include heavy sauces or gravies.

You can eat anywhere and diet! You may want to order only soup or appetizer and a salad and skip the meat portion of the meal. My wife and I enjoy a lovely restaurant where she has a shrimp cocktail and I have a crock of baked onion soup, and we then split a large Caesar salad. We can each enjoy a freshly baked hard roll, a salty bread stick, and a glass of white wine. Fresh fruit constitutes the dessert. We have spent a delightful evening and we've still had less than 1,000 calories each. You can dine out, eat this kind of restaurant meal, and stick to your diet. Just give up your snack for that day, and skip your meat portion for that evening.

Some of the meals that you might ordinarily eat in a restaurant can be prepared at home. They can be less fattening but just as tasty if a few slight changes are made in the ingredients. Don't be afraid to try new recipes. The recipe section at the back of this book includes exciting dishes that you can prepare with a minimum of trouble. Many ethnic foods are relatively low in meat and in fat, and they are not as difficult to prepare as you might expect. Try some Spanish rice; it contains about one ounce of lean meat per serving and is economical to serve. A hearty English meat stew with onions and carrots can be made without additional fats or oils by browning the meat first in a special nonstick pan.

Another surprise is that you can eat lasagna, especially at home. After you brown the ground meat, simply pour off the excess oil. Special cheeses, made with skim milk, are available. These have fewer calories and can be substituted for the regular cheeses. You'd be surprised that a diet dish can taste so good and still not add to your girth. Even spaghetti with meat sauce is acceptable on your diet. Remember to limit the quantities to a single serving (1 cup).

Create Indian curry recipes, or try Greek moussaka with eggplant, ground beef, and skim-milk cheese. High-protein meat substitutes made from soybeans or other vegetables are available. They can be used to extend ground meat, especially in Spanish rice, Indian curry, and in spaghetti sauce. They contain no additional fat.

Chinese cooking is usually low in meat. Chinese dishes focus on a variety of special vegetables, onions, chestnuts, bean sprouts, and rice. Using a steamer will enable you to serve crisper, more natural-looking, cooked vegetables. However, cornstarch-based sauces must constitute the cereal serving, and the amount must be limited. In general, it is the fat or oil of the sauce that adds extra calories.

Deprivation is not a feature of this diet. A sense of purpose is. Use the food-composition table in the Appendix to help educate yourself about the number of calories in various foods. Having a general idea of the caloric value of foods helps you plan menus and measure amounts of foods per serving. Remember, the more you know about food the more successfully you can diet. Trying new recipes will give you a sense of accomplishment and make the diet a more integral part of your life-style.

Become more adventurous. Some new kitchen equipment will make your new diet easier and more interesting. There are many new nonstick pots and pans, one of which provides a chemically treated surface upon which no sticking occurs. You can fry your low-cholesterol eggs without any butter, margarine, or shortening. You can even sauté vegetables in it without fat.

Other new kitchen aids you can look for include pasta makers, bread-dough mixers, and specially designed, inexpensive vegetable steamers. Your pasta can contain low-cholesterol eggs and less fat than the manufactured varieties. You can add vegetables like zucchini when you make your own bread. It is delicious and lower in calories. Steamers permit you to cook broccoli, carrots, and other vegetables and retain the nutrition, texture, and taste of garden-fresh vegetables. They help make the diet easier to follow.

A so-called new kitchen device—an unglazed clay pot—is similar to an ancient Roman casserole. Cooking foods in clay permits gradual heating of them without drying them out, and is excellent for fish, chicken, or beef. You can make delicious chicken with lemon, magnificently flavorful salmon, or a lavish beef Wellington with a little pastry, sliced mushrooms, and red wine. These alternative ways of cooking result in less fat, fewer calories, and often a more delicate flavor. The trick is to learn to consider diet cooking a challenge to your ingenuity and not a burdensome task.

This diet is a reaction to the well-established fact that most Americans eat much too much meat and saturated fat for their own good. Somehow the notion that potatoes, breads, and cereals are fattening, and well-marbled prime steaks are not, has been accepted as fact. It just is not true. It is difficult to follow a no-carbohydrate diet without developing symptoms of dietary deficiencies. In addition, removing carbohydrates from your diet clearly is meant to be a temporary phase of losing weight. Almost everyone will discontinue it eventually. As soon as you do, since you have learned nothing about how to eat, you'll resume your "good old ways" of eating and your weight will increase. I have many patients and friends who tell me they have lost hundreds of pounds on various quick diets, only to regain the weight as soon as they go off these diets. They don't understand that a lifetime commitment to a new dietary approach is their real salvation.

A forty-nine-year-old executive of a small company realized he had to lose weight. He went on a low-carbohydrate diet, ate little or no breakfast and almost no lunch. He had steak and cheese for supper and claims he lost twenty-one pounds, going from 194 pounds to 173 pounds in twenty-one days. I asked him why he didn't stay on the diet since he was clearly still overweight for his five-foot-nine frame. His reply was classic: "I felt terrible, my mouth felt like I had eaten cotton. I was dreaming constantly about eating a hard crisp roll, and I knew I could not stay on the diet for a long time." Both he and I are certain that he's gained weight since discontinuing the diet. He has dealt with the weight gain in a fairly typical way for ex-dieters. He refuses to weigh himself, preferring to relish the thought of his thin self at the weight of 173, despite the negative evidence he receives from his clothes and his eyes.

The truth is clear. You must be comfortable or you will not stick to any diet for any length of time. This diet is different! You'll experience no discomfort and you'll be able to persist.

The first forty-eight hours on the Natural Diet are very different from the so-called starvation regimes. You'll not believe you're on a diet. The breakfast and lunch menus are probably more liberal than your prediet breakfasts and lunches. The dinner will contain much less meat, but it is a small price to pay once you are determined to slim down. You'll be able to enjoy up to seven slices of bread a day, and all the green vegetables you wish. The liberal fruit allowance will satisfy your sweet tooth. It's unlikely that you'll have any sense of deprivation at all. You'll substitute greens and grains for meat. It will cost you less and you won't walk around like a hungry martyr.

Many people on a deprivation diet feel tired all the time. They can hardly keep on their feet. Some people have fainted on no-carbohydrate diets. Forget it! You'll experience no fatigue on this diet. Many people who are on diets find themselves taking a variety of medications. These include vitamin tablets and so-called appetite suppressants. Some dieters require drugs such as laxatives, because many diets do not provide enough food fiber. The Natural Diet is very different; there is no reason to take drugs for anything but *unrelated* medical problems.

Everyone on a diet *must* occasionally fall off the diet. Some dieters experience real guilt because of these very human foibles. This diet makes it easier to recover from backsliding. The truth is very simple: no one is perfect. The morning after an eating orgy you simply start over again with a good-sized breakfast, the one this diet outlines. Don't try to punish yourself by skipping breakfast and lunch the next day. It doesn't work. The volunteers who successfully followed this diet found that they could enjoy three full meals and a snack daily and still lose weight. So will you! The best protective measure you can take to avoid backsliding is to plan ahead. Even eating out or entertaining can be fun on this diet. Should you wind up on an eating spree, just chalk it up to experience and restart the diet the very next morning.

Many dieters believe incorrectly that enjoyment of food is impossible on a diet. Lots of delicious foods can be made lower in calories. Almost every food preference can be accommodated. You must simply tune in to a different way of eating, which does not mean eating less but does mean eating foods that are low in calories, learning how to prepare attractive dishes that do not abound in calories, and satisfying your sweet tooth with foods that are good for you.

Remember that cereals are the basis of most of the world's nutrition. There is a saying that a poor country has good bread and young prostitutes. Perhaps the economic deprivation means more pride and social investment in making the main source of nutrition (bread) more palatable. Certainly, ethnic breads such as rye, pumpernickel, pita, or tortillas are more fun to eat than typical enriched American white bread. One of the main points of the Natural Diet is that at any given time you can eat almost any food you enjoy—but you cannot have all of everything all the time.

Eating out at a party is not a major problem if you concentrate on the fruits and vegetables available and avoid the high-calorie dips. Given the situation of unlimited hors d'oeuvres, eat shrimp and tuna fish. At a formal sit-down meal, ask your hostess to give you a smaller portion of meat. If the meal is buffet style, it's easy for you to load up on salads and vegetables. Learn to enjoy bread or crackers without any spread. It's easier than you may think.

It is important for every dieter to keep from looking wrinkled and flabby while losing weight. Several things help to maintain the tone of your skin and muscles: exercise, gradual weight loss, avoidance of dehydration, and adequate nutrition. Exercise is crucial, even if it's a twenty- or thirty-minute walk once or twice a day (the next chapter goes into this in greater detail). Another important element is that weight should be lost gradually, not suddenly. Excessively rapid weight loss means that you lose muscle as well as fat. Many so-called authorities suggest that you fast—literally starve—as a method of weight control. If you are not strictly supervised, serious side effects can occur, some of which require hospitalization. It is much more sensible to plan on a gradual weight loss and a concurrent increase in activity. That's the way to avoid the wrinkled and flabby look. There is no need to look or feel drawn and worn on a diet. On this diet you'll look and feel younger!

Some people get colds, headaches, and tremors or shaky spells on crash diets. The simple truth is that they are malnourished. This need not be. The best diet you can follow is one that meets your needs for both weight loss and good daily nutrition. We've done the scientific calculations for you. All you need to do is eat, enjoy, and grow thinner.

Even a limited budget is not a problem on this diet. Several people on the diet noted that it lowered their total food bills. After all, meat causes the single most expensive dent in your food budget. The cereals of this diet, bread, beans, bagels, or breakfast cereals, are all relatively inexpensive. It is amazing that they are also better for you than the more expensive foodstuffs.

Vacations and holidays are important times for dieters and nondieters alike. These are the times we see family, friends, and food. You can have a vacation and still eat the foods you should. When you are entertaining others, you have more direct control over what is served. If you are eating out on a holiday, you'll soon adjust your patterns to accommodate the diet. Concentrating on cereals, fruits, and vegetables will get you through almost any party. If all else fails, and you simply must eat an ultra-rich meal because of a situation beyond your control, then simply relax and enjoy it. You'll be back on the Natural Diet *the next day,* and no single day's intake can completely ruin your dietary progress. Remember that you are in this for the long haul, so you can afford to be forgiving of your occasional lapses.

Up to 80 percent of the volunteers who lost weight on the Natural Diet maintained their weight loss six months later. Contrast that with the experiences of most dieters; only a handful manage to keep off the pounds. Very little has been published by fad-diet proponents about their long-term results. In Chapter 13 we will describe the research that documents that success of this diet. The best proof, of course, is your own experience. As you learn more about this dietary approach, you'll recognize that you can succeed in losing unwanted weight using these principles.

7.
Exercise

A man is as old as his arteries.

—Thomas Sydenham

The corollary to diet is exercise. Exercise is a necessary part of total physical fitness. Our muscles and bodies are designed to carry us to places and mobilize us for fight or flight. The Industrial Revolution marked the replacement of muscle energy by fossil energy. In our transition from muscle power to fossil power we gained cheap energy and the industrial age. We lost clean arteries and physical labor. It's time to turn back the clock a bit.

There are many reasons for increasing your physical activity as well as adhering to the Natural Diet. Physical activity is a method of releasing tension and keeping our muscles in tone and our skin flexible. Strength and endurance, the ability to work well and steadily, are increased by regular exercise. People who exercise regularly become more agile and more graceful. Because weight is a function of the total calories that we eat and the total amount of energy that we burn, exercise helps control weight. When we are in a positive balance—that is to say, we eat more than we burn—we gain weight. When we burn more calories than we eat, we lose weight.

Exercise does more than help control weight. Degenerative diseases like arthritis and diabetes and diseases of the heart and blood vessels are more common in the obese—especially in the physically inactive obese. Exercise lowers cholesterol and triglycerides. Over a period of time, exercise will help you lose weight. It will balance the tendency to gain weight as you grow older.

It is a good idea to learn the relationship between calories and exercise. It takes about 3,500 calories to gain or lose a pound of body fat. Walking a mile briskly will burn off approximately 100 calories. In order to burn off a pound of weight daily, you would have to walk thirty-five miles a day. Who can do that? However, if you walk a mile every day, you will lose a pound every thirty-five days, or approximately ten to twelve pounds a year. These figures imply no change in your eating habits. Adhering to the Natural Diet plus getting regular exercise will accelerate your weight loss and improve your overall physical fitness.

We all burn calories even when we sit quietly. Just by thinking, we burn about one calorie a minute, or sixty calories an hour. The actual number of calories burned is somewhat lower for women than for men. The difference is attributable to body size and weight, not sexual difference. Compare one hour of sitting quietly to these other activities: driving burns twice as many calories; walking slowly at two miles per hour, three times as many; riding a bicycle at about five miles an hour, four times; rowing or walking rapidly, five times; playing tennis, seven times the calories, or approximately 420 calories per hour. Volleyball, soccer, handball, and badminton burn ten calories a minute; skiing at five miles an hour and running at seven miles an hour burn twelve calories a minute. Clearly, such vigorous activities require a long period of training.

How much exercise do you need? At least thirty minutes a day! Some breathlessness after exercise is usual—in fact, desirable—but if you still feel sore or uncomfortable the next day, you have probably overdone it. Exercise should not interfere with your sleep. If you find that after vigorous activity you can't get to sleep, you probably exercised too much. Any fatigue and weakness that you do feel after exercise should be gone within an hour. If it is not, return to a lower level of exercise.

Exercising your large muscles (in legs, arms, shoulders, back, trunk and abdomen) helps build endurance. Running, swimming, and tennis are pleasant ways to use your large muscles. Do stretching exercises, twisting exercises, and bending exercises beforehand to improve your agility and muscle tone.

Start with two brief periods of about ten to twelve minutes a day, one in the morning and one in the evening. (Adjust these periods according to your age and activity pattern. Some may find a simple thirty- to forty-minute exercise period more convenient.) A brisk nightly walk is a good beginning. And remember that it is always necessary to check with your physician before beginning an exercise program.

Choose an exercise that is both pleasant and convenient. Clearly, activities such as tennis, hiking, handball, swimming, running, skiing, skating, and badminton are to be encouraged if they are available and interesting to you. If you have no specific sports interest, consider developing one.

Calisthenics are okay if you wish to do the most exercising over the shortest period of time, but they are routine and repetitive. The most successful exercise programs are those which you can integrate into your daily life. Encourage yourself to walk farther, climb stairs, and do the kinds of physical things that you ordinarily avoid.

Very few adults actually invest time and effort in regular, repetitive physical exercise. Of the 6½ million adults who jog, for example, only a third jog more than twice a week for more than ten minutes at a time. So only 2 million actually jog faithfully. Almost 50 million Americans do not engage in any physical activity that can rightly be called exercise. Of the millions of American men and women who do exercise, about 44 million walk; 18 million ride bicycles; 14 million swim; and 14 million do calisthenics. Once you accept that you must exercise regularly to look and feel your best, then you must plan a program. If exercise is not planned, it is usually not performed.

Lack of exercise is one of the most likely causes of the gradual weight gain that takes place in most adults. Participation in physical activities tends to decrease with age, but appetite tends to remain the same. This discrepancy leads to the accumulation of calories, and thereby, eventually, extra pounds.

In order to improve endurance, exercise has to be vigorous enough to place some stress on the cardiovascular system. Exercise should bring the pulse rate up to 70 percent of your theoretical maximum. The maximum pulse rate of the average individual is approximately 220 minus your age. For a forty-year-old healthy person, the maximum pulse rate would be 180, and 70 percent of 180 equals 126. These numbers are not exact. In order to check on whether you are exercising strenuously enough, take your pulse after exercising for one and a half to two minutes. Then compare your pulse rate to the theoretical maximum of your age. If you are not exercising enough to bring your pulse or heart rate to 70 percent of the maximum—or if it is way above—adjust accordingly. Unless an activity reaches a state of physical effort which requires the heart rate to approach 120, endurance does not improve.

Your personal exercise program will not cause a dramatic change in your appearance or feeling of fitness. Over a period of time, however, you will gradually note an improvement in energy, as well as endurance.

How much do you really know about exercise? Test your knowledge! Then I'll discuss the answers.

TRUE OR FALSE?

	T	F
1. You must exercise daily or it's a waste of effort.	—	—
2. Exercise programs must be started before you are twenty.	—	—
3. Always wear a vinyl or plastic sweatsuit when exercising.	—	—
4. Never drink water and always eat sugar before exercising.	—	—
5. Don't exercise in the noon sun when the temperature is in the nineties.	—	—
6. If you look good, you are in shape.	—	—
7. Exercise must hurt to be doing any good.	—	—

	T	F
8. Chest pain or light-headedness after a hard exercise session doesn't mean a thing.	—	—
9. After exercising, immediately jump into a hot shower.	—	—
10. You cannot exercise too strenuously.	—	—
11. After a heart attack you should never exercise.	—	—
12. Always do the same exercise.	—	—
13. Fat people can run longer distances than thin people.	—	—
14. Thirty-year-olds make better endurance runners than teen-agers.	—	—
15. Exercise increases your appetite.	—	—
16. It is wise to check with a physician before beginning an exercise program.	—	—
17. Muscles hurt during exercise because of "growing pains."	—	—
18. Tennis players make better lovers, but don't have sex before you compete.	—	—
19. Buying an exercise machine helps you exercise.	—	—
20. Only the athletically inclined can exercise.	—	—

Authorities are not in agreement about optimum exercise frequency. Many do believe, however, that exercises which use the large muscles are best for general fitness and weight loss. The large muscle masses of the legs, trunk, back, arms, shoulders, and abdomen require more caloric expenditure than the small muscles of the hands. Their usage promotes fitness by making more demands on the heart for an adequate blood supply. Some endurance exercises that use these mucles are running, jogging, swimming, walking, and competitive sports such as tennis, handball, squash, and basketball.

Exercise should be done at least three times a week. The best age to begin a regular exercise program is in the early teens. The age of ten is probably the best time, but it is unusual to find preteen-agers who are involved in a formal exercise program. Youngsters exercise, pleasurably and without planning, when they play games. Most middle-aged adults do not get very much exercise. But it is never too late to begin an exercise program. The age to begin an exercise program is the age when you decide to spend the time to improve your body.

A popular misconception is that it is best to wear clothing such as plastic suiting, which causes increased sweating and gives the illusion of more rapid weight loss. In reality, this merely encourages dehydration. The best clothing is comfortable and absorbent. Cotton is a favorite of those who do a great deal of exercise, but personal preferences certainly can be indulged by the large variety of leisure clothing that has been made available in recent years.

Many believe eating sugar just before exercises raises your level of energy, but this is unnecessary. Happily, the body's mechanisms maintain a near-normal blood sugar throughout all but the most vigorous exercise. Even patients who have diabetes can usually exercise without undo risk as long as they take some simple precautions. There is no harm in drinking water before exercise.

There is a saying that only mad dogs and Englishmen go out in the noonday sun. It is a good idea to avoid excessively vigorous activity on a very hot day, as this can tax your body unduly.

Some people assume that if they look good they are fit. This is far from true. Looking fit has a great deal to do with individual body build and how well your clothes are tailored. Real physical fitness is a function of performance.

Many people see exercise as a form of masochism. Rather, exercise should be looked at as a natural release of physical tensions and as a reward or diversion from other activities. If it hurts, you've overdone it.

After exercise, no one should feel either chest pain or light-headedness. It is amazing how often people accept these symptoms as normal: excessive shortness of breath is clearly an indication that you have done more than you should have.

It is not wise to stop abruptly after strenuous exercise. During exercise your heart beats rapidly and requires a large return of blood from the body in order to function normally. If you walk after strenuous exercise, the muscles' kneading action helps return blood from the legs to the heart by milking the veins. Should you suddenly come to a stop, blood will pool in your legs and you may have inadequate circulation through your brain. This may cause some light-headedness or even precipitate fainting (syncope).

A hot shower after a hard workout does not improve the circulation. In fact, it may further dilate the blood vessels and result in blood pooling. (This is the collection of blood in the veins which robs the heart of enough volume to pump out to the rest of the body. Because the blood stays in the veins, it is lost as far as your needs are concerned.) It is wise to delay having a shower after a hard workout until your cardiorespiratory system has returned to near normal.

Excessive shortness of breath or light-headedness at the time of the exercise or immediately thereafter means you've overdone it. You must compare your level of exercise with your usual activity. A sedentary person who has never done any exercise would be ill advised to run three miles on an initial workout. If you have been able to do two situps a day, or two chinups, and attempt to do twenty-five the next day, that would clearly be excessive. Some common sense is the most effective means to avoid trouble. You *can* exercise too strenuously.

People who have had heart attacks generally should avoid excessively strenuous activity during their initial recovery periods. With proper medical supervision they can and should gradually build up to rather vigorous activities. Many individuals who have experienced heart attacks have actually become long-distance runners. Like many of the other myths of physical activity, there is some ambiguity in Question 11. It is neither entirely false nor entirely true. But as a general rule, excessive strenuous activity can be a burden on an unprepared heart, and should be avoided, especially by cardiac patients.

It is not true that you have to stick to one type of exercise. In fact, if you do you are likely to become bored and quit. Your own preferences and your ability to work out your own schedule take precedence over what is written by authorities.

Some believe that fat people who have stored up additional calories should be able to run longer distances than normal people. This is false; actually fat people require more energy and oxygen to run the same distance because they are carrying a heavier weight.

Interestingly enough, thirty-year-olds make better endurance runners than teen-agers. Certainly younger people are better at sprinting, but age does seem to have some advantages. (Maurice Chevalier, when asked if he objected to growing older, once replied, "It's not bad if you consider the only alternative.")

Exercise does not increase your appetite. Another myth is that exercise requires more protein foods. Calories adequate for the energy you need when you exercise can be provided by carbohydrates or body fats. Exercise does increase your well-being; and some people may even notice that they have less of an appetite after exercise.

Always check with your doctor before beginning any exercise program. Medical supervision is necessary to determine exactly how much exercise your body can tolerate and benefit from. If an examination reveals that there is a potential problem, the doctor can advise you on how to limit the exercise you take so that it will be beneficial, not dangerous. A good initial medical checkup should include a complete physical examination, an electrocardiogram, and determination of blood cholesterol and triglyceride values after a twelve-hour overnight fast.

It is not true that muscles may hurt during exercise because of "growing pains." There is no such thing as a growing pain.

Many people believe that they should avoid sexual intercourse before athletics. While this is clearly a personal matter, it has not been demonstrated that sexual activity will prevent you from performing well in some other athletic event. A well-trained person is likely to have less cardiac acceleration and less shortness of breath during intercourse. If being physically fit does not make you sexier, it at least makes you more comfortable in sexual performance.

Exercise machines are not necessary. They may enrich the manufacturer and salesperson, but they are not valuable to most dieters. Most of these devices gather dust after the initial fervor wears off.

Everyone needs exercise, whether one is athletic or not. Basically, what it all boils down to is this: being in condition gives us the ability to do more—more work and more play. Fitness requires exercise which will slowly develop your muscles. Fitness clearly will help you achieve and maintain your best weight.

You needn't worry about becoming a muscle-bound Amazon or Charles Atlas. Exercise will not make you a competitor for the Mr. or Mrs. Universe title.

SELECTED EXERCISES

The following group of exercises are useful in developing and maintaining fitness. For each you should start off counting slowly so you can develop a regular rhythm. Count aloud, one digit a second, until your rhythm is well established.

Abdominal Head and Shoulder Curl

1. Lie on your back with your legs straight and your arms at your sides. 2. Slowly raise your head and shoulders off the floor. 3. Hold and count to five. 4. Return to starting position.

Repeat ten times, gradually and slowly increasing the repetition rate.

Standing Reaching Bend

1. Stand erect with your feet comfortably apart, arms extended over your head. 2. Stretch as high as you can, keeping your heels on the ground. 3. Hold the position for ten or fifteen counts. 4. Return to starting position. 5. Slowly bend forward and touch the ground, keeping your knees straight. 6. If you cannot touch the floor, reach as far down as you can.

Start with five repetitions and gradually increase the number you perform.

Sit-up with Arms Crossed

1. Lie on your back with your arms crossed on your chest, hands grasping opposite shoulders. 2. Slowly rise to a sitting position. Keeping your knees bent will make this exercise easier. The exercise can also be performed with your knees straight and your arms out. 3. Lie down again slowly, keeping your legs straight out in front of you.

Start with five repetitions and gradually increase.

Shoulder Horizontal Arm Circles

1. Stand erect with arms extended sideways, palms facing upward. 2. Make six-inch circles backward with arms. 3. After fifteen or twenty circles, reverse. 4. Turn palms downward and do circles forward.

Gradually increase the number of complete circles in both directions.

Push-ups

1. Starting position is lying prone, hands outside of shoulders, fingers pointing forward, with the knees bent. (Beginners should start with their knees bent and their feet touching the floor, supported by their hands outside their

shoulders.) 2. Straighten arms, keeping back straight. 3. Return to starting position.

Start with one or two and very gradually increase the number you do; aim for ten to twenty.

Side Leg Lifts

1. Lie on your right side with legs extended and hands over your head. 2. Slowly raise left leg as high as possible. 3. Lower left leg to floor. Do ten repetitions.

Roll over on left side. 1. Raise the right leg as high as possible. 2. Lower the right leg. Do another ten repetitions.

Heel Raises

1. Stand erect hands on hips, feet together. 2. Raise the body onto the toes. 3. Return to starting position.

Do fifteen repetitions.

Sit-ups

1. Lie on back with arms at sides and legs extended. 2. Sit up, extending arms toward the feet. 3. Slowly lie back to starting position.

Start with five repetitions and gradually increase aiming for twenty.

Quarter Knee Bends

Starting position: stand erect, hands on hips, legs comfortably spaced. Count 1: bend knees to forty-five-degree angle with heels on the floor. Count 2: return to starting position.

Repeat twenty times.

Forward Bend

Stand erect, feet shoulder-width apart, knees flexed; keep hands on hips. Action: slowly bend trunk forward and down, keeping knees flexed. Count 2: return to starting position.

Repeat ten times.

Straddle Hops

Stand erect, hands on hips, feet together. Count 1: jump to side-straddle position with feet spread shoulder-width apart. Count 2: return to starting position.

Start with five and gradually build up, aiming for twenty-five repetitions.

Running in Place

Stand erect, arms at sides. Action: run in place with feet and knees pointed straight ahead.

Begin with five minutes; gradually increase to ten to fifteen minutes, if you are comfortable and have been cleared to run a mile by your own physician.

8.

Nutrition Is Not a Dirty Word

Many more people by gluttony are slain
Than in battle or in fight, or with other pain.

—Anon.

Nutrition means different things to different people. To some, nutrition is a special diet. To a physician, it is a way of dealing with the sick. To a biochemist, it may be a complex organic chemical reaction. To a politician, it is perhaps a campaign issue. To food faddists, it is almost mystical.

Good nutrition means good health. Good nutrition helps build resistance to infection, assures proper growth and development, and aids in the repair of the body. Good nutrition prevents deficiency diseases. Well-nourished people are healthy, vigorous people; they are not overweight. Good nutrition insures healthy teeth and skin, and normal energy and endurance.

Conversely, poor nutrition inhibits growth, causes undesirable changes in weight, flabby muscles, and dry skin. Poorly nourished people are listless, easily fatigued, susceptible to infections, and recover more slowly from illnesses. Poorly nourished people have short attention spans and are often apathetic, depressed, and irritable. Extreme examples of this are found in the accounts of the survivors of Nazi concentration camps and in the writer Solzhenitsyn's description of the hunger in the Russian prison camps; purposefully inadequate and poorly balanced nutrition were part of the torture. In an attempt to lose weight, many well-motivated but misinformed people subject themselves to unnecessary physical and mental stress, believing that only starvation produces weight loss. *Not true.* You need not starve on the Natural Diet.

Starvation denies you the pleasure of eating. Not only will you feel psychologically deprived, you will be *physically* deprived. Fad diets fail because they cannot succeed. Unbalanced diets cannot be continued indefinitely without damaging health and well-being. You need proteins, minerals, vitamins, water, carbohydrates, and fats to maintain a healthy, well-nourished, ideal-weight body.

In order to provide yourself with the good nutrition necessary for good health, you must understand what makes a diet good and why. The efficient working of the human body depends on adequate supplies of various substances. Once you understand how the body works, it will be easier for you to provide it with what it needs.

CARBOHYDRATES

It is a myth that carbohydrates are more fattening than other foods. All foods are chemical compounds, the composition of which determines the calories. Carbohydrates are composed of three elements: carbon, hydrogen, and oxygen. Carbohydrates contain twice as much hydrogen as oxygen. In plants, carbohydrates are produced by the process of photosynthesis; sunshine transforms carbon dioxide (CO_2) to sugar or starch.

There are several types of carbohydrates. Simple sugars include fructose and galactose. Glucose is the type of sugar found in the blood; it nourishes the brain and the heart. Double sugars include sucrose, which we know as table sugar.

Complex carbohydrates include starch, which is found in grains, vegetables, and bananas, and glycogen, which is found in animal liver and muscle. Cellulose, another complex carbohydrate, is found in the bran of cereal grains and in the skins and fibers of fruits and vegetables. In the United States, about half of the caloric intake is carbohydrate. In the Orient, where rice is the leading staple food, most calories are provided by carbohydrates. Wheat is the staple cereal in Russia, Western Europe, India, and the United States. Corn and beans are preferred in Central and Latin America. Not all carbohydrates are sweet; complex carbohydrates—starches—are bland.

Grains, fruits, vegetables, milk, and concentrated sweets provide carbohydrates. Some whole grains of wheat, corn, rice, oats, rye, barley, buckwheat, and millet contain protein, minerals, and vitamins. Since certain losses do occur in the processing of grains, most manufacturers have enriched the flours they produce with thiamin, riboflavin, niacin, and iron. By 1962, more than 90 percent of the white bread sold in the United States was enriched. Today, one slice contains, on the average, three grams protein, one gram fat, and eighteen grams carbohydrates.

By emphasizing cereals and increasing the proportion of carbohydrates in the diet, we are stepping back through history to an earlier, less affluent time. In the last sixty years the proportion of carbohydrates in the American diet has decreased significantly. We have increased our intake of fat and protein; the incidence of cardiovascular disease has also increased.

Carbohydrates supply energy to support the metabolic processes and the heat the body needs. We are warm-blooded animals and if we do not burn enough carbohydrates, we have to burn fat or protein or we will perish. Carbohydrates are cheap and universally available.

Perhaps the diets of early agricultural societies were superior to the affluent diet of today. The Natural Diet will provide a healthy alternative for those who follow it, gaining some of the advantages of "the good old days."

PROTEIN

Proteins are complex substances. Like carbohydrates, they contain carbon, hydrogen, and oxygen. But in addition, they contain nitrogen, and some contain sulfur and phosphorus. Occasionally copper, manganese, and zinc are found in proteins. Proteins are found in all living things: plants, animals, even bacteria. All tissues contain protein. Protein is 16 percent nitrogen and contains various arrangements of amino acids.

In adults, the protein requirement is fairly stable at nine-tenths of a gram per kilogram (half a gram per pound) of body weight, or about forty-five to sixty-five grams (about two ounces), depending upon body weight. A popular misconception is that more protein is required for heavier labor: it is not. The additional calories needed are supplied by carbohydrates and fats. Proteins are required in the body because there is a constant need to replace worn-out body cells. There are thirty-two amino acids. The body produces all but eight of them by itself; therefore, we must provide those eight in the foods we eat.

A balanced diet provides adequate protein for all body needs. Dietary proteins are provided by eggs, milk, cheese, cereal grains, and flours, as well as meat, fish, and poultry. Nuts, seeds, fruits, and vegetables contain varying amounts of protein. In the United States, meats, fish, and poultry contribute about 33 percent of the protein we eat. Cereal grains provide 30 percent and eggs and cheese provide 25 percent. Vegetables provide about 10 percent of our protein supply and nuts the remainder. A variety of different protein foods provide for diversity as well as a balanced protein intake.

Protein is needed to provide adequate numbers of new red blood cells, so that anemia does not occur. Proteins are also necessary to produce antibodies, which fight disease. Proteins contain four calories of energy per gram. If the diet contains much more protein than is needed, the excess protein is burned or stored as fat. When the diet does not contain sufficient calories, part of the body's protein will be utilized for energy rather than building or replacing tissues.

Proteins are not magic; they are vital but often misunderstood. The use of high-protein fad diets without carbohydrates means that some of the excess protein will be burned for energy instead of carbohydrates. This is usually an expensive way to provide energy. Protein in excess of normal requirements is usually unnecessary and wasted.

FATS

Lipids are fats composed of carbon, hydrogen, and oxygen. These are the same elements that are found in carbohydrates. Fats, however, contain a smaller proportion of oxygen. When fats are burned they provide nine calories per gram, or more than twice as much energy as proteins or carbohydrates.

Most fats are insoluble in water. *Saturation* describes the amount of additional space available for hydrogen in the fat. Saturated fatty acids cannot accept additional hydrogen; unsaturated fatty acids can. A polyunsaturated fatty acid is one in which two or more double bonds are present. Unsaturated fats help reduce cholesterol. Bonds are the connections which bind various atoms together in a molecule. In fats, many of these connections are occupied by atoms of hydrogen. Some fats have unused bonds which could contain additional hydrogen atoms, but which do not because of their so-called unsaturated structure. Polyunsaturated merely means several connections are not filled with hydrogen atoms. It is not known why unsaturated fats affect the level of blood cholesterol.

Fats are found in both animal and vegetable sources. Foods rich in saturated fats include whole milk, cream, ice cream, cheese, egg yolk, fatty meats (beef, lamb, pork, ham, bacon), coconut oil, salt pork, chocolate, cake, cookies, pie, and rich puddings. Polyunsaturated fats are found in vegetable oils, especially safflower, corn, cottonseed, soybean, sesame, and sunflower oil. Some salad dressings and special margarines are made with polyunsaturated fats. Salmon, tuna, and herring contain polyunsaturated fats.

Fat helps maintain body temperature by providing insulation underneath the skin. This insulation is clearly more attractive in certain areas of the body than others. Some individuals are too well insulated from the outside world. Fats in the diet help you feel full. Fats add flavor and palatability to food.

Cholesterol is an important chemical. Its significance is far greater than the proportion of the total fat intake it represents. Cholesterol is a white, waxy substance not unlike fat but with a different chemical structure. It is found in foods such as egg yolk, liver, kidney, brains, and shellfish. Animal fats such as beef, pork, milk, cheese, ice cream, butter, and cream are all cholesterol rich. A high cholesterol count increases the risk of heart disease, though a certain amount of cholesterol is necessary for good health. My research has demonstrated a relationship between the progress of heart disease and lipid levels.

Most ordinary fats contain triglycerides, which are combinations of glycerol and three fatty acids. High levels of triglycerides increase the risk of heart disease, but the increase is less marked than for cholesterol. Triglyceride levels fluctuate with nutritional states. To measure triglycerides, the patient must fast for twelve to fourteen hours. Fasting is less important for cholesterol measurements. An easy way to decide if your physician has measured your triglycerides is to recall whether you were told to fast for twelve hours before blood tests were taken. If fasting was not required, the chances are that you've never had a triglyceride determination done.

We all eat various amounts of cholesterol. An average adult man consumes 600 to 700 milligrams of cholesterol per day. An egg contains about 250 milligrams of cholesterol, four ounces of meat contain about 80 milligrams, sixteen ounces of whole milk contain fifty milligrams of cholesterol, and two tablespoons of butter contain seventy-five. Ideally, no diet should include more than 100 to 200 milligrams of cholesterol a day. There is no risk of cholesterol deficiency, since the liver can manufacture all that is required for normal sexual functions.

Most of us eat about 40 percent of our calories as fat, which is probably excessive. There has been much discussion and disagreement about the role of fat in heart disease. Currently, reduction in both fat and cholesterol appear prudent (see Chapter 11). Some people inherit a tendency toward high cholesterol and/or triglycerides. Change in diet may be less useful for these few people.

WATER

Most of us do not think of it as a nutrient, but water is absolutely necessary for survival. About two-thirds of body weight is water; blood is mostly water. Every cell in the body contains water. Muscle contains as much as 80 percent water and bone about 25 percent.

Water carries body wastes to the kidneys, serves as a lubricant, and helps regulate body temperature through evaporation.

Ordinarily we lose water every day through our kidneys, skin, lungs, and bowels, but most is lost in the urine. The daily water requirement is about one milliliter per calorie, or about two quarts a day. Almost any beverage is largely water. We also manufacture about a fourth of the water we need through oxidation of carbohydrates, protein, and fat. Solid foods such as cheese, meats, fruits, and vegetables supply another fourth.

The amount we lose depends on the amount we take in. In the absence of kidney disease, water intake and output are regulated almost automatically. Some water is lost every time we exhale or perspire.

MINERALS

Minerals (salts) are inorganic substances, and very different from protein, fats, and carbohydrates. Minerals combine with protein to form compounds necessary for life processes.

Some minerals are found in extremely small amounts in the body. Calcium is the mineral found in the largest amount, specifically in the bones and teeth, which it helps make stronger. The calcium in the bones is not fixed there, but can be withdrawn and used for other purposes. Calcium is also found in body fluids, where it speeds blood coagulation and transmission of nerve impulses, and regulates the heartbeat. Calcium deficiency only becomes evident after many years of inadequate diet. Milk and milk products, hard cheeses, and cottage cheese are the major sources of calcium; alternative sources are broccoli, cabbage, cauliflower, oranges, canned salmon, oysters, lobster, and dried beans.

Phosphorus is another required mineral. It interacts with calcium, especially in the bones and teeth, and helps regulate the absorption and transportation of fats. It is found in all cells and is important to normal muscle function. Phosphorus helps regulate the acidity of the blood, and is contained in enzymes (chemicals which speed body reaction), which regulate energy metabolism. Phosphorus is found in milk, pork, fish, turkey, peanuts, chicken, and beef.

There are only about five grams (one-sixth ounce) of iron in the body, but iron is an extremely important mineral. Iron is used in the production of hemoglobin, which carries oxygen to all parts of the body. Iron is also found in muscle tissue. Healthy women require about twice as much iron as men because they lose iron with normal menstruation. Meat, dark-green leafy vegetables, beans, nuts, and enriched flour, bread, and cereal are good sources.

Iodine is important to thyroid function, and helps prevent some forms of goiter. Iodine is found in iodized salt, some seafood, and vegetables grown in soil rich in iodine.

Magnesium, found in bones and teeth, helps to regulate irritability and muscle contraction. It is contained in some of the enzymes needed for energy. Magnesium is found in chlorophyll of green leafy vegetables, nuts, cereal grains, and seafood. Magnesium deficiency is not likely to occur without some type of malabsorption, chronic alcoholism, or uncontrolled diabetes.

Salt (sodium chloride) is also important, although most of us consume far more than is required. Certain diseases, especially heart disease and high blood pressure, are treated by reducing the amount of salt in the diet.

Potassium is found in all cells. Most foods supply plenty of potassium, and dietary deficiency of this mineral does not occur.

Trace elements are required for very specific purposes. Fluorine helps protect the teeth; it is best supplied in drinking water. Chromium affects carbohydrate metabolism, but deficiencies of chromium do not appear in the absence of other disease. Chromium is found in corn, whole grain cereals, and meat. Cobalt, a constituent of vitamin B^{12}, is essential to normal cell function and is necessary to the nervous system. It is found in liver, kidney, milk, and grains. Copper, a catalyst used in the production of blood pigment (hemoglobin), is found especially in the liver, brain, heart, and kidney. Liver, shellfish, whole grains, poultry, and nuts supply copper. Manganese is also necessary for certain enzyme systems and blood formation. It is found in whole grains, beet greens, nuts, fruits, and tea. It is unlikely that manganese deficiency occurs in humans. By and large trace minerals, while important, are very seldom the cause of deficiency disease in an affluent society.

VITAMINS

The discovery of vitamins marked a great improvement in nutrition. Although they are present in the body in very small amounts, their effect on the treatment of deficiency diseases has been little short of miraculous.

Misunderstanding of the function and use of vitamins is almost universal. The popular press would have you believe that vitamins produce miraculous effects in a healthy body. In actuality, vitamins are organic compounds that are essential to specific metabolic reactions for life and growth, but they do not provide energy. They do make it possible for the body to use nutrients in a more effective way. Vitamins function as part of enzymes. (Enzymes are organic materials produced by living cells, but which act independently of the cells. They tend to speed a reaction, but are not themselves altered by it.)

It is convenient to divide vitamins into two groups: one, fat-soluble vitamins, which includes vitamins A, D, E, and K; and another, water-soluble vitamins, which includes B-complex vitamins and vitamin C. Vitamin A was the first fat-soluble vitamin to be identified. Vitamin A helps the eyes see in dim light. It helps maintain the skin, the integrity of the lining of the mouth and nose, and helps in normal bone and tooth formation. The daily adult requirement for vitamin A is 5,000 units. Vitamin A is found in liver, in green, yellow, and dark-green leafy vegetables, and in cantaloupe, apricots, fortified margarine, whole milk, egg yolk, and cod and halibut fish oils.

Vitamin D prevents rickets, a bone disease, and helps the body use calcium and phosphorus to build and maintain strong bones and teeth, and promote normal growth. An intake of 400 units of vitamin D is necessary daily. Vitamin D is found in butter, cream, egg yolk, liver, fish liver oils, and fortified milk. Salmon, tuna, and sardines are also sources of vitamin D.

Vitamin E is a fat-soluble vitamin whose role is poorly understood. It has enjoyed an enormous popularity in recent years because it is alleged to cure heart disease and improve sexual function. There is no good scientific evidence for either claim. Vitamin E is found in many foods, especially salad oils, margarine, whole grain cereals, nuts, green leafy vegetables, and legumes. Deficiency of vitamin E is probably not a problem in humans. Since vitamin E is widely available from common foodstuffs, supplemental vitamin E does not appear necessary.

Vitamin K helps promote normal blood clotting. It is found in green leafy vegetables. Vitamin K can also be synthesized by bacteria in the bowel. There is no need to take supplements, except for certain bleeding disorders.

Vitamin C, ascorbic acid, is a water-soluble vitamin, essential to building the cementing material that holds the cells and tissues together. Lack of vitamin C causes scurvy. This disease is romantically described in records of the sea journeys of sixteenth-century explorers. The discovery of the effectiveness of citrus fruit as a cure for scurvy is attributed to a British naval physician. Vitamin C also aids in normal bone and tooth formation and in the healing of wounds. It helps the body use iron and resist infection. A minimum intake of ten milligrams of ascorbic acid a day will prevent scurvy. Today, scurvy is seen only in alcoholics or food faddists who avoid all natural sources of vitamin C. Sources of ascorbic acid include citrus fruits, leafy vegetables, tomatoes, strawberries, cantaloupe, cabbage, and green peppers. Whether vitamin C aids in the prevention or treatment of colds is still open to debate. If it is effective, the dosage recommended for the prevention of colds far exceeds the minimum daily requirement.

The B-complex vitamins are also water soluble. Vitamin B^1 is also called thiamine. It promotes normal appetite and digestion, helps convert carbohydrates into food energy, and maintains the integrity of the healthy nervous system. Deficiency causes arrested growth and beriberi, which is marked by symptoms in the heart and nervous system. Thiamine is present in whole cereal grains, nuts, beans, and some meats. Much of the thiamine that is lost in the milling of wheat flour is replaced when the flour is enriched. Enriched cereals provide a good source of vitamin B^1. The recommended allowance for thiamine is between one-and-a-half and two-and-a-half milligrams a day. Thiamine is the one vitamin which may be deficient in an average diet.

Riboflavin or vitamin B^2 is another water-soluble vitamin of the B complex It helps the body use oxygen, and promotes healthy skin and eyes. The recommended amount for an adult is 1.7 milligrams per day. Riboflavin is present in milk, liver, heart, kidney, lean meats, dark-green vegetables, dried beans, almonds, and enriched breads and cereals.

Niacin or "nicotinic acid" is another B-complex vitamin, the deficiency of which causes pellagra. Pellagra affects the skin and the nervous system. Niacin is found in tuna, liver, lean meats, fish, poultry, peanuts, whole grain, enriched or fortified breads, cereals, and peas. Brewer's yeast is also a good source of niacin. Corn products contain some niacin. The daily requirement of niacin is about fifteen milligrams.

Vitamin B^6 helps the body use protein. It helps use carbohydrate and fat for energy and helps keep the skin and nervous system healthy. Vitamin B^6 is found in pork, liver, heart, kidney, milk, whole grain and enriched cereals, wheat germ, yellow corn, and bananas. The daily recommended amount of vitamin B^6 is approximately two milligrams a day.

Other vitamins in this series include pantothenic acid, which is necessary for carbohydrate, fat, and protein metabolism. Ten milligrams a day is the recommended adult requirement, and deficiency diseases are not likely since it is widely found in natural foods. Vitamin B^{12} is a vitamin which aids in the formation of normal red blood cells. It is found in liver, kidney, milk, fish, eggs, cheese, and meat. The RDA (recommended daily allowance) is six micrograms a day. This is easily available in a diet which contains normal amounts of protein.

Notice how often cereal grains supply the essential nutrients. Cereal grains are an economical, nutritious source of calories, minerals, and vitamins. An awareness of proper nutrition is more important to a dieter than to those who eat without restrictions. Good nutrition presupposes knowledge, but is easily accomplished on the Natural Diet. Moreover, there is no reason to take supplemental vitamins because vitamins are more appropriately supplied by the natural foods included in this diet. The important thing to realize is that good nutrition demands a lifelong commitment.

9.

Carbohydrates, Villain or Victim?

To lengthen thy life, lessen thy meals.

—Benjamin Franklin

Most people are misinformed about sugar, carbohydrates, and "empty" calories—calories that occur in foods that supposedly have no nutritive value. Many food faddists, believing that sugar is uniformly bad, classify all carbohydrates as empty calories. Nothing could be further from the truth. Since calories are a measure of the amount of food energy in a given foodstuff, they represent an important source of nutrition. When we ingest more calories than we can use, we store the extra calories as fat. These extra calories can come from sugars and starch, and often do. Sugar and starch are fattening when they are eaten in excess, but in no way are they more fattening than equivalent excesses of fat, protein, alcohol, or "natural food." Many fad diets blame sugar and starchy foods for obesity. Since carbohydrates contain four calories per gram, they are much less fattening than an equivalent amount of fat, which contains nine calories per gram. Alcohol contains approximately seven calories per gram, and so is more "fattening" than sugar or starch.

While it is true that some people are unable to control their intake of calories unless they keep carbohydrate foods at a minimum, such so-called "carboholics" are rare and are analogous to alcoholics. About 4 percent of the population is alcoholic, yet the vast majority of us can enjoy an occasional drink without suffering an uncontrollable urge to drink ourselves to oblivion. Similarly, the vast majority of normal people can and do eat carbohydrates without losing control.

87

The popular myth of "empty" calories assumes that starches and sugars are useless. By overemphasizing protein and fat, they actually advocate an unbalanced diet. Excessive restriction of carbohydrates is not necessary for weight control. Starches and sugar are inexpensive and pleasurable sources of calories. We all need energy to maintain body heat, to carry on day-to-day activity, and to nourish our hearts and our brains. Total avoidance of carbohydrates leads to the production of *ketones,* which are by-products of fat metabolism. This so-called ketosis, which is fervently desired by a popular low-carbohydrate diet, often causes nausea, lack of well-being, and dehydration.

Those who resolve to diet often make false starts by omitting certain foods (sugars and starches) entirely, or by concentrating on very few food products as their only source of nutrition. Some diets focus on eggs, or grapefruit, or bananas, or steak, or even alcohol. Over a long term, they are neither balanced nor do they provide enough diversity. These restrictive diets eventually fail because the initial self-deprivation that they call for approaches martyrdom and the menus are so dull that they eventually become intolerable.

Carbohydrate-restricted diets are expensive, unimaginative, and tend to be very high in fat. Indeed, the usual protein foods such as meat and cheese have a very high proportion of fat calories. In fact, they usually contain more fat calories than protein calories. Thus the steak, meat, and egg diets are, by definition, high-fat diets. Many people lose weight on these diets and attribute it to the mysterious—actually nonexistent—"fat-mobilizing factor," whose proponents hold that fat calories are burned more quickly than sugar calories. Yet it is *absolute caloric reduction* and *fluid shifts* which account for the weight loss. Unless you eat less, you cannot lose weight. Balance among carbohydrate, fat, and protein in the diet is important. The continued control of the amount of total calories in relation to exercise determines the success or failure of weight control.

It is misleading to assume that only foods containing vitamins and minerals are desirable. In terms of their weight, the amount of vitamins and minerals required in a healthy diet is extremely small. Excesses of vitamins and minerals do not improve health; indeed, serious injury can be caused by excessive intake of some vitamins, especially fat-soluble ones.

Many earlier diets took great delight in attacking sugar as a specific evil. Indeed, certain publications listing the nutritional rating of foods have imposed a negative value on foods containing refined sugar. As a source of energy, however, sugar is perfectly adequate. Sugar meets energy needs; proteins meet rebuilding needs.

Some people claim that purified carbohydrates, especially sugar, contribute to disease, specifically coronary disease. This theory has received considerable public attention, but there is little evidence to support direct association between a high sugar intake and the development of coronary problems. The incidence of heart disease has increased in the last fifty years; sugar consumption has not. Obviously, factors other than sugar account for the observed increase.

Sugar has another virtue: it is an inexpensive source of calories. It takes much less land to grow the food that provides calories from sugar than that for cereals, chicken, or beef. About 0.15 acres of land will produce 1 million calories of sugar; it takes 1.2 acres of land to produce 1 million calories from wheat as refined wheat flour and 0.9 acres of land to produce 1 million calories of wheat as whole wheat flour. It takes two acres of land to produce a million calories from hogs, including both pork and lard, and 9.3 acres of land to produce a million calories from chickens. In light of the American love for beef, it is interesting to note that no less than seventeen acres of land are required to produce a million calories from steers. It is apparent that more than 100 times as much land is required for the equivalent caloric production of beef as of sugar.

Moreover, carbohydrates contribute no cholesterol or saturated fat to the diet. Increased cholesterol intake is much more likely to cause heart disease than increased sugar intake. In experiments, sugar does not cause arteriosclerosis in animals: fat and cholesterol do.

Based on this data, it becomes obvious that a successful, healthful diet is a well-balanced diet. You will not lose weight by adhering single-mindedly to a fad diet that eliminates essential nutrients from your food intake; bolstering a fad diet with vitamin pills will not solve the problem. To achieve long-term weight loss, a balanced diet is a must—a diet that contains carbohydrates as well as proteins, sugar as well as fat. The key is reduced amounts and increased exercise.

10.

Popular Misconceptions about Losing Weight

Excessive eating is like deadly poison to the human body, and is the root of all disease.
—Maimonides

PHYSICAL CONDITIONS

When you know the facts, dieting is less difficult. One of the most frequent dietary misconceptions is that glandular (endocrine) or thyroid problems cause obesity. Many obese patients are unnecessarily treated with thyroid extract or wrongly convince themselves that an underactive thyroid is causing their overweight condition. The number of patients who are hypothyroid and obese is really remarkably small. Indeed, many people with thyroid disease are not overweight. Those who are overweight need both thyroid medication *and* fewer calories to achieve a normal weight.

Another common myth is that low blood sugar (hypoglycemia) is a common cause of obesity. Not true. It *is* true that many obese people will demonstrate hypoglycemia on a glucose tolerance test (which is a test of periodic blood sugar levels after a standard load of glucose), but the hypoglycemia is not the cause of the obesity. More likely it is the other way round. Patients who have significant hypoglycemia are often quite thin, and the addition of relatively small amounts of carbohydrate when symptoms surface suffices to control the problem. Much has been made of this problem in popular publications, but recent medical studies have demonstrated that many patients have hypoglycemia without any apparent symptoms. Rarely is hypoglycemia a life-threatening condition. It is often used as a glib explanation of nonspecific neurotic symptoms. It does not cause obesity in the majority of people with weight problems.

HEREDITY

Another old wives' tale is that obesity is hereditary. While people may have fat relatives, relatives do not cause fat. Your relatives may entice you to eat more, but the calories, not the relatives, make you fat. Many people gain weight eating the same amount of food that just sustains their thin friends. This seems puzzling until you analyze their physical activity and the efficiency of their gastrointestinal tracts in absorbing fats. When individuals are compared, there are minor but significant differences in how they go about their activities and how they absorb the calories that they eat. These factors explain much previously inexplicable obesity in those who truthfully believe that they eat less than their thin friends.

An example might be useful. Assume that you are unfortunate enough to absorb fats at a 10 percent greater rate than your closest friend. If you are both on a daily diet containing 100 grams of fat, you would tend to retain ninety more fat calories than your friend. In a year, this would be about 35,000 calories or ten pounds of fat a year, without overeating. Since most obesity results from the prolonged accumulation of extra calories, you can see that minor shifts in fat absorption can account for obesity. It is incorrect to brand every obese person a glutton.

"FAT" FOODS

Many people believe that only certain foods turn to fat and others are unrelated to obesity. This is, unfortunately, not the case. The body is able to change carbohydrates and proteins into smaller chemical units, called two carbon chains. Using these two carbon building blocks, the body can then build fat. It is possible to produce fat out of any food that you eat, but *the fat will only be deposited if the number of calories taken in exceeds the energy requirements of your body* at a particular time. So it is not a question of having a particular food turn to fat, but rather of taking in too much food. A calorie is a calorie, regardless of its source.

GOING TO EXTREMES

There is no end to the self-flagellation of the obese person who wishes to lose weight. Sometimes, obese people are told to fast—starve—but not to death. Fasting and starving are similar; despite semantic differences, they both involve stress and nutritional deprivation. Also, there are radical operative "solutions" which involve the surgical shunting of part of the small intestine by a bypass procedure. True, this will decrease the absorption of calories, but it is dangerous. It can cause uncontrolled diarrhea, and may even result in death. While surgical bypass may occasionally be useful in morbid obesity (obesity of more than double normal body weight or a minimum of 100 pounds of excess weight), it is inappropriate for people with more usual weight problems. Bypass is a research procedure. The casual use of either starvation or surgical bypass should be condemned.

SKIPPING MEALS

A favorite pseudodiet is skipping meals. Many people, especially fat ones, are willing to skip breakfast and skimp on lunch. Unfortunately, "dinner" can then begin at six P.M. and end at bedtime. Studies of animals have already shown that if an animal eats a specific number of calories on a one-meal-a-day basis, it will store more fat than if it consumes the same amount of calories in five feedings spread out over a day. So nibbling has its practical and psychological advantages. But if you are dieting and nibble ten times a day, it means that you must think "I've had enough!" ten times a day. A better compromise is three scheduled meals and a late-night snack.

Unfortunately, you do not benefit from skipping meals. In addition to the poor nutrition that you subject your body to, there is good evidence that people who skip breakfast and drink black coffee for lunch merely eat a larger evening meal. This not only makes for more discomfort, but probably deposits even more fat. It can also cause subtle defects in how the body handles calories and carbohydrates. Obese people often eat most of their calories after six P.M. The most commonly skipped meal, unfortunately, is breakfast—and there are distinct disadvantages to skipping breakfast. These include fatigue in the later morning hours, less adequate performance, and an increased likelihood of a ravenous appetite in the evening.

DRUGS

Many people believe that they can eat whatever they want as long as their physician supplies them with a variety of drugs, especially amphetamines (stimulants to the central nervous system), which presumably help them lose weight. These drugs have significant toxic effects and contribute little more than placebo (fake sugar pill) value in permanent weight reduction. Many studies have failed to show the consistent effectiveness of these drugs. Where the drugs have been used in controlled experiments, it is apparent that the patients who receive placebos also lose weight, although at a somewhat slower rate. It is probably the relationship to the physician, as counselor, and the discipline of a research project that provide motivation to control eating, not the drugs.

I conducted an interesting study on the effectiveness of a new diet pill. The drug was a harmless derivative of cellulose, which swelled to many times its original volume when exposed to water. Before eating, the dieter would take several tablets with a glass of water. The pills would swell and partially fill the stomach so the dieter would feel full sooner, eat less, and lose weight. This research was carefully planned; another group of volunteers received inert tablets. Both groups lost weight during the study, but the cellulose group lost only slightly more. The weight loss in the group taking the inert tablets must be attributed to the interest of both the volunteers and the physician in the program.

SPECIAL FOODS

Many people falsely believe that they can reduce the number of calories by toasting bread or washing rice. This is purposeless, unless you prefer the taste. Some food substitutions, such as skim milk, diet margarine, and no-calorie soft drinks, *do* make a difference.

Some high-protein foods, especially meat, have been thought useful in dieting because they burn up calories in the process of digestion. This is scientifically correct. The phenomenon called "specific dynamic action" refers to the caloric cost of the breakdown and buildup of the component blocks of the protein as it is utilized by the body. However, it accounts for little more than 10 percent of the protein calories. Most meats contain a high proportion of fat, and to eat more protein in order to lose weight is self-defeating. Pure protein is only available in the laboratory or as egg white, and probably tastes the way it sounds. So most protein foods are fattening, despite specific dynamic action.

Everything we eat has calories; and although the number of calories is fewer in certain foodstuffs such as green leafy vegetables, there is no free lunch. Fad diets promise something for nothing, implying that the patient will lose a lot of weight in a very short time. This effectively disregards the first law of thermodynamics: The first law of thermodynamics, more commonly known as the law of conservation of energy, states that the total energy content of a closed system is constant. If the total amount of energy is constant, energy cannot be created or destroyed, but energy may be converted from one form to another. If energy (i.e., calories) is ingested, it must be burned, stored, or excreted. If you eat more and/or burn less, you will gain energy (i.e., weight.) The supposed weight loss in a fad diet is only a temporary water loss. True obesity is not resolved by water shifts, but only by the loss of body tissue, especially fat.

Carbohydrate diets, although they are popular, have no special virtue to recommend them, but are merely simplistic approaches to the chronic problem of obesity. The fact remains that even the Natural Diet functions because of the interdependence of various foodstuffs. A good balanced diet provides the kinds of variety and interest that permit you to follow the diet long enough to attain your ideal weight. Fad diets do not provide accurate information on nutrition. When you return to "normal" eating, you are very likely to regain all of the weight you lost, since you have not established any patterns of eating that are at all different from those that caused you to become obese originally. By concentrating on cereals at all four meals (an appetizing, satisfying diet, low in fat and sufficiently low in calories), you can lose weight pleasantly and safely. The low cost could even help reverse obesity among those with low incomes.

DIETING WITHOUT RESULTS

Some people cannot believe they will lose weight by dieting. Painfully slow weight loss is often puzzling to the physician and frustrating to the dieter. Sometimes it is simply due to failure to follow the diet. Many people conveniently forget what they have eaten. Some dieters incorrectly believe that a simple potato or a slice of bread will add pounds of fat, but that they can eat unlimited quantities of steak. Some dieters are simply dishonest and choose not to reveal their indiscretions.

This entire matter has been thoroughly investigated. From 8,000 women who were members of various diet clubs, twenty-nine were selected for a further study. They had been dieting for an average of fifteen months and had previously lost an average of fifty pounds. The volunteers were all taken to an isolated country house where they were closely supervised. All baggage was searched on arrival to insure that no food was smuggled in. The patients were permitted walks on the grounds only when accompanied by a staff member.

A 1,500-calorie diet was provided, and all food eaten and wasted was measured. All but nine patients lost weight in the three weeks of the research study. Some of the nine lost between one and two pounds and might have lost more if the study had been continued beyond three weeks. Some were shorter than sixty inches, and 1,500 calories was simply too much for them. Some were clearly too inactive, and had very low rates of metabolism. Finally, we were left with perhaps one or two who did not lose weight because their bodies adapted to the low-calorie diet (an extremely rare phenomenon). The short, inactive woman who is not very far from her ideal weight is likely to have the greatest difficulty achieving weight loss.

Contrary to myth, calories do count. There are no revolutions in diet, but new nutritional information is accumulating. The water, grapefruit, and drinking man's diets are simplistic. You can purchase a variety of belts, pulleys, pads, machines, and nonabsorbent sweat suits, but they are not worth their cost. Only caloric reduction can help you lose weight over the long haul. Ideal weight and vigorous good health require a nutritionally balanced diet. The Natural Diet will help you achieve these goals.

11.

Natural Diet,
Atherosclerosis, and Heart Disease

They have digged their grave with their teeth.

—Thomas Adam

Hardening of the arteries (arteriosclerosis) results from atherosclerosis, a degenerative process characterized by the accumulation of a fatty, mushy, yellow material in the inner wall of an artery. The term *atherosclerosis* is derived from *athere*, the Greek word for mush. The inner wall of the artery becomes encrusted with an irregular deposit called *atheroma*, which contains cholesterol. Much as a muddy river builds up deposits along its banks, the arterial passageway gradually narrows and blood flow through the artery is obstructed. Traditionally this process has been considered a normal one in old age, but in actuality it need not develop.

Atherosclerosis is a complex process. The rate of its development varies enormously in individuals and among different population groups. Atherosclerosis is a long-range process which produces no symptoms for a considerable period of time. It is only after this process has significantly interfered with the flow of blood through the arteries that symptoms develop. An interference with the blood supply to vital organs can occur, and the symptoms depend on which organ is affected and to what degree. Obstruction of the arteries to the brain and heart is most critical. Obstruction of the blood vessels to the extremities and the kidneys is somewhat less likely to cause dramatic, life-threatening catastrophies.

Coronary artery disease is the major unresolved health problem of Western society. Every year approximately one million Americans experience either acute heart attack (myocardial infarction) or sudden death due to an interference with the flow of blood through the coronary arteries. Myocardial infarction means the death of part of the heart wall. Interference in the blood flow may cause either no symptoms or minimal symptoms, or it may lead to myocardial infarction. Narrowing of the *coronary arteries* is a form of heart disease that kills and disables thousands of young men. More men than women are involved. Middle-aged men in the United States suffer from one of the highest coronary death rates in the world. There has been a little progress recently in reducing these high death rates. An average man, selected at random, has a 20 percent (one in five) chance of developing significant coronary disease before he is sixty. This most often occurs as a heart attack, but occasionally it takes other forms.

Another classic form of heart disease, *angina pectoris,* is characterized by squeezing chest pain underneath the breastbone. Lack of oxygenated blood causes the pain because the heart muscle is deprived of oxygen. Angina lasts only a few moments and does not cause permanent damage to the heart. It is usually brought on by emotional stress, exertion, hurrying, eating a heavy meal, or a combination of these. A *heart attack,* or an acute episode of abnormal heart functioning, means there has been death of part of the wall of the heart. The amount of destruction depends on how much heart muscle has died for lack of oxygenated blood. If the damaged area is very small, then full recovery can eventually occur. The area around the destroyed muscle is surrounded by only partially damaged muscle, and in time this muscle can recover.

Once coronary disease due to atherosclerosis has developed, the outlook is far from attractive. About 25 percent of the people who have a heart attack die within three hours, often because they do not understand the significance of the pain. Some people die before they can reach the hospital or obtain adequate medical care. Another 10 to 15 percent will die within the first several months after discharge from the hospital. The risk of death among those who do recover and return home is approximately five times that of an unselected age-matched population. Given these bleak statistics, it seems obvious that our efforts must be concentrated on primary prevention. It is only by preventing or controlling the atherosclerotic process that the disabling effects can be mitigated. Control of vascular disease requires modification of many habits, especially dietary.

Many studies have been made on the possibility of predicting whether a person is likely to develop coronary disease. Various risk factors have been identified and their significance, taken individually and in combination, has been extensively researched. The most significant and potentially reversible risk factors are elevated blood levels of cholesterol, triglycerides, and sugar; cigarette smoking; high blood pressure (hypertension); certain personality traits; obesity; and lack of exercise. Some risk factors can be altered; others, such as one's sex and family history of heart disease, cannot.

You may believe that a reduction in your blood fats is not important. You may even have been told that your cholesterol count is normal. The concept of *normal* deserves further comment. The normal serum cholesterol level is usually between 150 and 250 milligrams per 100 milliliters of blood. (These values of serum cholesterol apply to healthy individuals.) There is very good evidence, however, that these levels, although they are considered normal, are nevertheless higher than desirable.

Most people in other countries have considerably lower cholesterol levels. They also have a much lower risk of cardiovascular disease, especially for men over forty. It may well be that lower cholesterol levels reduce the risk of heart disease. The Framingham study, begun in Massachusetts in 1948 and continued for twenty-five years, involved 5,000 volunteers. These volunteers (originally all free of disease) were examined and tested every two years. Some developed heart disease and some did not. The study revealed that the risk of coronary disease in men was mathematically related to their cholesterol levels. Patients with cholesterol levels above 260 milligrams, usually considered a "high normal" in the United States, had four times as many heart attacks as those whose cholesterol count was below 200 milligrams. If 200 and 260 milligrams are both normal, obviously the lower level is more desirable. All other things being equal, this diet should help you lower your cholesterol.

Arteriosclerotic lesions (injuries) can be induced in laboratory animals. This experimentally produced arteriosclerosis permits scientists to study ways of controlling and reversing the disease. The first experiments producing arterial lesions in a rabbit were those done by N. Ignatowski, a Russian, in 1908. Interestingly enough, Ignatowski fed the animals meat, milk, and eggs—the major components of the diet of many Americans. This experiment has been repeated informally in men, women, and children all over the Western world over the last sixty years under the guise of "eating well." N. Anitschkow, also Russian, extended Ignatowski's work; he fed rabbits pure cholesterol in dissolved vegetable oil. He demonstrated both a rise in serum cholesterol and the production of cholesterol-containing yellow patches in the arterial wall.

Note that these arteriosclerotic lesions were produced experimentally in animals by modification of the diet to include more cholesterol and fat. In general, it is not possible to produce atherosclerotic lesions in animals without doing this.

With very few exceptions, people whose diets are high in saturated fats and cholesterol have elevated serum cholesterol levels, and high incidence rates and mortality rates from premature heart disease. People whose diets are low in cholesterol and saturated fats tend to have low mean cholesterol values, and a low incidence of and mortality from premature heart disease. In a given population, the risk of developing premature heart disease from coronary artery narrowing rises as the serum cholesterol rises. This relationship, which has been documented in American men, between the level of cholesterol and the incidence of atherosclerotic coronary disease, is continuous. While there is no absolute critical level which separates high- and low-risk people, coronary artery disease is very rare among those who have a serum cholesterol under 180 milligrams per 100 milliliters of blood. Cigarette smoking, high blood pressure, and glucose intolerance (inability to tolerate normal amounts of sugar without large blood sugar rises) also increase the risk of coronary heart disease.

Data from the Framingham study showed that in a forty-year-old man who had a normal electrocardiogram (a recording of heart activity), a cholesterol level of 185 milligrams percent, normal blood sugar, did not smoke cigarettes, and had a blood pressure of 105 systolic (i.e., pressure when the heart contracts), the risk of developing coronary heart disease in a six-year period was less than 0.7 percent. This would rise over the next twelve years, but would still be quite low, considering the low starting point.

Contrast this lucky man with his forty-year-old neighbor who feels perfectly well. He has a cholesterol count of 335 milligrams percent, a systolic blood pressure of 195, smokes cigarettes, has an elevated amount of blood sugar, and minor changes in his electrocardiogram. This unfortunate man falls into a group with a 37.1 percent risk of developing coronary disease in six years—fifty times as high a risk as the first man. The statistics also imply that within twelve to eighteen years almost everyone in the second category will suffer from coronary artery disease. Provided that some simple risk factors are properly evaluated, it is possible to predict, with a reasonable degree of accuracy, who will develop coronary disease. Keep in mind, however, that although statistical risks are correctly applied to large populations and can aid in the medical treatment of individuals, they do not provide exact data about the future of an individual. Individual variations must always be taken into consideration.

Nevertheless, the prudent approach is to try to reduce the risk factors in your own life. Knowing an individual's smoking, blood pressure, electrocardiogram, and blood sugar patterns permits concentration on those who are the highest risks. Dietary management to reduce cholesterol and triglycerides is an approach which is readily available and inexpensive. The Natural Diet results in lowered intake of lipids or fats; the greatest reduction is usually seen in those whose cholesterol counts are highest. The corresponding weight loss helps normalize blood sugar and blood pressure.

In an international atherosclerosis project, data from all over the world was pooled to compare the amount of atherosclerosis in aortas. (The aorta is the main blood vessel leading from the heart, which nourishes most of the body through its many branches, including the coronary arteries.) Information about 31,000 aortas was collected between 1960 and 1965 in fifteen large cities throughout the world. The severity of the atherosclerosis observed varied markedly in different locations. In general, people in countries where the intake of saturated fat and cholesterol was high had more severe atherosclerotic lesions in both the aorta and the coronary arteries than did populations with low fat intake and low serum cholesterol levels.

In a recent study which measured mortality rates in twenty-two developed countries, the mortality rates of middle-aged men from coronary disease showed sizable differences. These differences corresponded to differences in nutrition, such as daily calorie intake and saturated fat and cholesterol levels. The United States had the unenviable position of being at or near the top of the list in cholesterol and saturated fat levels, and, predictably, in mortality.

In another extensive study, blood samples were taken from people in seven different countries: Finland, Greece, Italy, Japan, the Netherlands, the United States, and Yugoslavia. Twelve thousand men aged forty to fifty-nine were studied for ten years or more. Middle-aged American men had four times as many heart attacks as men from Greece, Japan, and Yugoslavia. The highest five-year incidence rates were recorded in men from eastern Finland and from the United States, where, respectively, rates of 120 and eighty cases of heart disease per 1,000 people were recorded. In contrast, the five-year incidence rate for coronary disease in Crete, Dalmatia, and Japan was twenty or less per 1,000 people. Since the studies all used the same criteria, the observed differences were not due to diagnostic variability, or lack of skilled physicians.

In a study published in the *New York State Journal of Medicine,* I reviewed the role of lipids in the progression of heart disease. Fifty-eight patients who had had repeated coronary angiograms were examined. It was possible to measure the progression of existing coronary atherosclerosis in these patients. The risk factors, including high blood pressure, diabetes, cigarette smoking, and elevated cholesterol and triglycerides, were examined. In comparing those whose disease progressed (i.e., became worse or more occluded) and those whose did not, only the presence of excessive blood lipids was statistically significant. While this is a preliminary report, it may provide a clue to reducing the rate of progression in preexisting coronary disease by control of blood lipids.

Additional information has been derived from studies of populations whose diets have changed. During World War I, observations suggested a decline in atherosclerotic disease among German civilians. This was attributed to a decreased fat and calorie content in their diet. These observations were reinforced during World War II, especially in countries where food shortage was acute. Where people decreased their fat and caloric consumption, there was a corresponding decrease in coronary disease. After the war, incidence of coronary disease increased as diets higher in fat and calories became more readily available.

Shifts of population other than during wartime can also mean substantial changes in diet. There have been several such shifts which permit observations on the relationship between diet and disease. Yemenite men were observed when they first migrated to Israel in 1948 and for the next twenty-five years. There is little doubt that the longer they lived in Israel, the more their incidence of heart disease rose. In Yemen, these men had a very low fat intake, and very few of them developed coronary disease. When they migrated to Israel they gradually increased their fat intake, and the incidence of coronary disease in their population rose dramatically.

Similarly, it was found that Japanese people who migrated to the United States developed higher serum lipids and more coronary disease than native Japanese. Clearly, factors other than dietary manipulation are involved, but the studies do provide suggestive evidence for the relationship between diet and heart disease.

The first rule for being healthy must be to care for your body. The reduction of cholesterol and fat that you will achieve by adhering to the Natural Diet is safe. Elevated serum cholesterol *is* a real risk, and *now* is the time to do something about it.

12.

Can We Reverse or
Delay Atherosclerosis?

Feed sparingly and defy the physician.

—John Ray

Overeating can cause atherosclerosis and coronary artery disease; there is a link between the dietary lipids (cholesterol, triglycerides, and saturated fat) and atherosclerosis. Can the lowering of elevated serum cholesterol and triglyceride levels reduce the incidence of coronary disease? Will we thereby halt the progression of coronary atherosclerosis? Is it likely that regression of already established coronary athersclerosis is possible? I believe the answer to all three questions is yes.

While the causes of atherosclerosis are unknown, one theory suggests that the introduction of cholesterol from the circulating blood plasma into the inner wall (intima) of the coronary arteries accompanies atherosclerosis. The deposition of cholesterol and the formation of blood vessel lipid accumulations or *atheroma* (a raised collection of cholesterol and scar tissue within the inner lining of an arterial wall) are not uniform. If they were, disease would be predictable. Since they are not uniform, the disease and its symptoms are unpredictable. It is more likely to occur at bends, angles, and branchings in blood vessels. In theory, elevated blood cholesterol increases the deposits in the inner wall. Can a marked lowering of cholesterol reverse this process? If it can, then atherosclerosis can be reversed. The evidence is hopeful.

In rabbits on a high cholesterol diet who developed atherosclerotic deposits, regression has been effected by lowering the dietary intake of cholesterol. Studies done with monkeys show actual reduction in the narrowing caused by atherosclerosis; change in diet caused the reduction. The evidence that the lesions can be modified in monkeys provides some support for a similar reversibility in humans. Recently, drugs which lower cholesterol have also been shown to reverse coronary artery disease in monkeys.

There have been three somewhat similar studies done with humans. In a New York City "Anti-Coronary Club" study, patients modified their diets to lower their cholesterol levels. They were encouraged to increase the amount of polyunsaturated fat in their meals. These people were not institutionalized; they cooked at home, ate out, and went to parties. Two other studies were done in institutions: one in Los Angeles among veterans living in domiciliary facilities; another in Helsinki, Finland, comparing the male populations of two mental hospitals. In each of these studies there was a decrease in the incidence of new heart attacks in the experimental (cholesterol-lowering) group as compared to the control (normal unmodified food intake) group. In the Los Angeles study, the decrease in the incidence of heart attacks was most pronounced in men under sixty-five and in men who had had the highest values for cholesterol prior to the initiation of the study. All three studies evidenced some reduction in the incidence of coronary disease among people whose diets were modified to reduce cholesterol intake.

Another study combined a low-cholesterol diet and supervised exercise. Blood-vessel narrowing decreased. A recent development is very exciting. A new technique that measures whether the fatty deposits inside arteries are becoming larger or smaller can document regression of atherosclerosis. It is a safe, repeatable technique. Now we can prove that treatment with diet and drugs can reverse atherosclerosis.

Antithetical experiments have caused atherosclerosis by raising cholesterol levels. Such experiments have been conducted repeatedly with animals. A recent report of a cardiac transplant patient witnessed a similar unfortunate effect in a human. The patient was a fifty-eight-year-old man who received a twenty-four-year-old's heart. (The donor had died from a brain hemorrhage and had a normal heart.) The patient died nineteen months after the transplant. At the autopsy it could be seen that he had extensive atherosclerosis of every coronary artery. Even the aortic portions of the transplanted heart, which had been inspected prior to the surgery and were known to be normal, were markedly involved. The recipient had a cholesterol count chronically above 300 milligrams percent due both to diet and to genetic level. This case demonstrates the speed with which atherosclerosis can progress. It is one more bit of evidence implicating cholesterol in the cause and progression of atherosclerosis.

In a recent study, I examined patients who had coronary artery disease. All the patients had had coronary angiograms done twice, a year or more apart. It was possible to identify those whose arteriosclerotic narrowing did not progress. They were in the minority; the natural history of the disease is one of relentless progression. Those whose disease did not progress were likely to have lower cholesterol levels.

What has not been proved yet is whether coronary artery disease is reversible in humans after aggressive treatment to lower the cholesterol level to below 200 milligrams percent. Studies currently under way may provide such proof. (My current study of patients who have undergone saphenous vein bypass surgery for coronary artery disease may shed some light on this.)

So there is evidence that atherosclerosis in humans can be reversed. Although the results are encouraging, the studies are inconclusive. Certain statistical flaws such as high rates of dropout and the absence of absolutely suitable control groups tend to reduce the reliability of these studies. However, using the information currently at hand, we can design a diet which should help lower the lipids and thereby prevent or delay coronary disease. Such a diet should be low in cholesterol, animal and saturated fats, and total calories, and have adequate but not excessive sugar and sufficient fiber.

The Natural Diet as proposed in this book meets these qualifications admirably. Although many people, including some physicians, feel that the evidence is not sufficient to justify dietary modification by healthy people, most health professionals do accept the need for risk reduction in high-risk individuals. If we, healthy individuals included, do not act on the information provided by these extensive though incomplete studies, then we risk permitting nature to take its course. And since there is no danger in such action on the part of healthy individuals, it can only be helpful to institute these dietary changes.

The meal plan on page 110 illustrates the amount of cholesterol in a day's food intake on the Natural Diet. The total cholesterol intake is, at most, 130 milligrams.

Saul Bellow, in his book *Humboldt's Gift,* quotes Samuel Daniel as saying, "While timorous knowledge stands considering, audacious ignorance hath done the deed." Clearly waiting for the final *i* to be dotted and *t* to be crossed results in the loss of opportunities, perhaps of lives.

Presumably conflicting theories of cholesterol's impact on atherosclerosis will be resolved after the completion of extensive cholesterol-lowering studies. It may take a decade before the final answers are in. Clearly, it makes sense to act on the information already available. The history of medicine is replete with old fogies who preached caution in the face of every therapeutic advance.

Conclusive evidence that the treatment of high blood pressure results in decreased morbidity and mortality has been available only for the last ten years. Hypertensive patients, who were denied treatment until the final documentation of its effectiveness, paid for that delay in strokes, congestive heart failure, and death from kidney failure.

Not all elevated serum lipids are due to dietary excess. There is a small

ONE-DAY MEAL PLAN SHOWING CHOLESTEROL INTAKE

Meal	Serving	Cholesterol (mg.)
Breakfast		
Fruit	1 serving	0
Breads and		
cereals	2 servings	0
Milk, skim	1 cup	5
Lunch		
Meat	2 oz.	48
Breads and starch	2 servings	0
A vegetable	As desired	0
Fat, unsaturated	1 serving	0
Fruit	1 serving	0
Dinner		
Meat	3 oz.	72
Breads and starch	2 servings	0
A vegetable	As desired	0
Fat, unsaturated	1 serving	0
Fruit	1 serving	0
Snack		
Milk, skim	1 cup	5
Bread and starch	1 serving	0

Sources: *Central New York Diet Manual*, Central New York Dietetic Association, 1973; and *Planning Fat Controlled Diets*, Colorado Heart Association.

minority of Americans who have severe hyperlipidemia which is genetic (inherited) rather than environmental. These rare individuals do show some improvement in their cholesterol and triglyceride levels when they adhere to special diets, but they also require more aggressive treatment.

The vast majority of Americans who develop coronary heart disease do not have genetic hyperlipidemia. Their moderate cholesterol and triglyceride levels are often thought to be normal or borderline. Nevertheless, they are more likely to develop coronary heart disease than people with low blood lipids. Anyone can reduce cholesterol intake by having a diet that contains less than 130 milligrams cholesterol and is low in saturated fat. Anyone on the Natural Diet will reduce cholesterol level, risk of coronary heart disease, and weight.

13.

Results of Natural Diet Research

Hunger:

Not only the best cook, but the best physician.
—Peter Attenberg

The teacher of the arts and the inspirer of invention.
—Persius

The worst political advisor.
—Albert Einstein

The mother of fascism.
—Joseph Gould

Despite the numerous claims of allegedly successful diets which have appeared in both lay and professional publications, the results of treatment for obesity have been discouraging. Many reports of diet treatment are poorly documented. One of the better studies described a group of 200 obese patients who were initially hospitalized to initiate diet therapy and were then followed as outpatients for one year. All lost some weight in the hospital on a calorically restricted diet. On follow-up after one year, only 12 percent had maintained at least a twenty-pound weight loss and only one of the 200 had achieved ideal weight—despite the cost and inconvenience of the initial hospitalization. Other studies have reported equally bleak statistics. Fad diets, behavior modification, psychotherapy, and various drugs have all been proclaimed as individually effective, but the fact remains that the vast majority of obese people have been and continue to be unsuccessful dieters.

Dieting is not usually considered a hazardous procedure. Nevertheless, as I have pointed out earlier in this book, some high-fat, low-carbohydrate diets are clearly ketogenic (ketosis results from the incomplete metabolism of fatty acids), raising acidity in the blood and resulting in elevation of both cholesterol and triglyceride values. Low-carbohydrate diets may also cause dehydration. Other diets are so poor nutritionally that deficiency diseases would occur if patients were to follow them religiously. Some of the young people who adhere to the Zen macrobiotic diet have developed malnutrition, scurvy, and anemia.

Some stressful fad diets precipitate a variety of psychological and nervous symptoms. A distinctive night-eating syndrome is called *nocturnal hyperphagia* (eating more than 25 percent of total daily calories after the evening meal.) Insomnia and morning anorexia (loss of appetite) are often symptoms of this condition. Such patients experience a high incidence of psychic complications, including neurasthenia, severe anxiety, and even psychotic depression. Some dieters develop weakness, restlessness, nausea, difficulty in concentration, and apathy.

Twenty-six hospital employees volunteered to follow the Natural Diet and have their weight and lipid changes recorded. The criteria for participating in the eight-week study were an initial weight 10 percent or more above ideal, a nutritional interview and assessment, and a review of family history of disease and eating patterns. All patients' fasting cholesterol and triglyceride values were measured. The patients agreed to keep a daily food intake record (diet diary), to be weighed weekly, and to have a fasting cholesterol and triglyceride level measured at the end of eight weeks. All subjects continued all their work and home responsibilities.

As you will recall, this research diet is a low-saturated-fat, low-cholesterol, exchange-system diet in which items in each food group may be freely exchanged for each other. It supplies 130 to 160 grams of carbohydrate, sixty-five grams of protein, forty grams of fat, and an average cholesterol intake of 115 to 130 milligrams per day. The diet's 1,260 daily calories are distributed as follows: approximately 50 percent carbohydrates, 30 percent fats, and 20 percent proteins.

The participants were given an expanded list of breads, cereals, and starches that could be incorporated into their meals. The exchange system and the use of a diet diary were explained. The dieters attended several lectures on nutrition and the role of exercise. We did not attempt to police the participants; adherence to the program was voluntary.

The ages of the volunteers ranged from nineteen to sixty-three years; the average age was forty-four years. There were twenty-three women and three men. There was a positive family history of diabetes in ten people, cardiovascular disease in nine, and obesity in seventeen. All were well enough to continue their full work program.

A common comment of the subjects on this diet was that there was too much food in the breakfast and lunch. This reflects the inadequate breakfast and tiny lunch habits of many people, especially those who eat at night. Interestingly, despite the frequent statement "I can't lose weight on any diet containing over 1,000 calories," all but one subject lost weight on this diet. While most admitted an occasional indiscretion, adherence to the diet was generally good.

There was a mean weight loss of fifteen pounds, with a range from −35 to +2 pounds. The weight loss was sustained: a follow-up at six months showed that twenty of twenty-four had maintained their weight loss (two were lost to follow-up).

WEIGHT LOSS ON NATURAL DIET (IN POUNDS)

Subject Number	Initial Weight	Final Weight	Weight Loss
1	199	188	11
2	216	202	14
3	158	147	11
4	177	157	20
5	176	166	10
6	177	161	16
7	198	183	15
8	209	199	10
9	151	138	13
10	202	186	16
11	136	129	7
12	138	131	7
13	176	172	4
14	140	135	5
15	197	185	12
16	212	201	11
17	152	143	9
18	241	220	21
19	158	143	15
20	193	178	15
21	262	227	35
22	254	247	7
23	178	174	4
24	174	162	12
25	137	130	7
26	148	150	+2

The treatment of hypercholesteremia and hyperlipidemia with appropriate dietary modifications is documented as well. In our study, the average cholesterol level fell from 243 mg. percent to 220 mg. percent and the mean triglyceride level fell from 146 to 130 mg. per 100 milliliters of blood.

Predietary cholesterol and triglyceride levels were classified as: (1) ideal—cholesterol less than 200 mg. percent and triglyceride less than 100 mg. percent; (2) normal—cholesterol 201−240 mg. percent, triglyceride 101−150 mg. percent; (3) abnormal—cholesterol greater than 241 mg. percent and triglyceride greater than 150 mg. percent. This group began with a mean

CHOLESTEROL CHANGES OBSERVED ON NATURAL DIET

Subject Number	Cholesterol Range (Mg. %)	Mean Before Diet	Mean After Diet	Mean Change (Mg. %)	(% Change)
2	Less than 200	194	190	4	-2
12	201–240	222	209	13	-6
12	241 or above	273	236	37	-14
26	All values	243	220	23	-10

TRIGLYCERIDE CHANGES OBSERVED ON NATURAL DIET

Subject Number	Triglyceride Range	Initial Value	Final Value	Change	% Change
8	Values under 100	67	73	+6	+9
11	101–150	128	136	+8	+6
7	151–+	265	185	-80	-30
26	All values	141	130	-11	-8

elevated cholesterol level of 273 mg. percent and dropped to a mean of 236 mg. percent—a 14 percent reduction. The elevated triglyceride mean fell from 265 to 185 mg. percent or 30 percent. These drops are in the same range as can be obtained using hypolipidemic drugs, but without the attendant problems of toxicity and cost. Minor individual increases in triglyceride means were seen among those with initially low levels. These ranged from 6 to 8 percent and did not raise any previously normal values to the elevated level. These increases do not appear to have clinical significance.

At the end of eight weeks, most subjects felt more pride and confidence in themselves because of their weight loss. They generally felt better and were less fatigued. In comparison to other diets that they had tried, the volunteers agreed that the experimental diet was more satisfying, easier to follow, and caused less hunger. The dieters especially liked the wide variety of food choices, the ease in adapting the diet to regular family food patterns, and the diet's economy.

Serum lipid levels which have been heretofore considered normal or average are associated with an increased risk for coronary artery disease (CAD). It is possible to relate the progress of coronary artery disease to lipid levels when levels in the ideal range (cholesterol 200, triglyceride 100) are considered. Recent data from Dr. David Blakenhorn of the University of California Medical School and my own studies have demonstrated a relationship of lipid values to progression and regression of CAD.

This study demonstrated that outpatient volunteers can successfully lose weight on this Natural Diet (which is relatively high in carbohydrates). It was well tolerated by the dieters, who registered lowered serum cholesterol and triglyceride values.

14.

Fiber—Facts and Fantasy

Ye shall eat the fat of the land.

—Genesis

Even today, Ponce de Leon would have no trouble selling his Fountain of Youth. People want to believe in quick miracles. Recently, claims have been made about the properties of dietary fiber that are not unlike the claims of the snake-oil merchants of the Old West. Despite claims to the contrary, fiber does not save your life, nor does it significantly reduce an elevated cholesterol level. Fiber may be fine, but it is not a panacea, despite its good press.

Fiber is indigestible carbohydrate material which is composed of filaments and gives strength and support to plant tissue. Fiber is present in most foodstuffs, but is found most abundantly in natural cereal grains, fruits, and vegetables. Fiber is also found in oregano, curry powder, and parsley. Bran, the outer protective covering of a wheat kernel, consists of cellulose and other fiber materials which go through the intestinal tract virtually unchanged by the digestive process. By absorbing large amounts of water, fiber adds bulk to the food in the lower bowel and eases elimination. Fiber is not found in meat or dairy products. The only reasonable advocacy of fiber diets is in the treatment of constipation and diverticulosis.

Diverticulosis is a bowel disease of adult life evidenced by multiple small outpockets (diverticula) that are found in the large intestines, usually in people who are over forty. Some patients with diverticulosis have no symptoms at all, while others suffer abdominal pain, constipation, or diarrhea. Diverticulosis is rare in Africa and Asia. Its rarity is now attributed to high-fiber diets. A

123

high incidence of diverticulosis occurred in England about the time improved milling methods (which remove most of the fiber from flour) developed. At one time the standard approach to the treatment of diverticulosis was a low-fiber diet. In recent years medical authorities have reversed the recommended treatment.

Some authorities have even suggested that appendicitis, varicose veins, phlebitis, and diabetes are causally related to lack of fiber in the diet. Such theories are based on studies done in southern Africa, where the natives eat large amounts of fiber in the form of bran. These natives are much less prone to develop diverticulosis, diabetes, cancer of the colon, excessive cholesterol, and heart disease than are affluent Americans. So goes the myth. It is supported only by population studies, not by hard evidence.

As the West grew affluent, grain became less important in the diet as other foods became more available. Increasingly, Americans have become meat-eaters, and grain is largely fed to cattle. What grain we do eat is usually milled and converted into white flour; the outer husks of the wheat (bran) are discarded. All this makes the standard American diet practically fiber free.

What is well documented already is that an increase of fiber in the diet will help avoid constipation. Enthusiasts who take in large amounts of bran in addition to the fiber normally found in a balanced diet will notice an increase in the bulk of their stools. These two effects are the only proven effects of additional bran or fiber in the diet.

The effect of fiber on hemorrhoids, varicose veins, and phlebitis is speculative at best. No studies have yet convinced most authorities that fiber lowers the incidence of cancer of the colon.

A leading baker has recently marketed a deliberately fiber-enriched bread that contains powdered cellulose, which increases fiber content and reduces the calories. This bread has 25 percent fewer calories per slice than ordinary enriched bread. The question of how many people will enjoy eating a bread mixed with an extract of wood pulp has not been answered yet. During the siege of Leningrad, the Russians did use sawdust to make their black bread go further. So we know that starving people will eat bread laced with sawdust. But will affluent Americans pay premium prices for bread laced with powdered cellulose?

Additional fiber means more elimination from the bowel, certainly a happy circumstance for those who are afflicted with constipation. Many people, however, find increased gas and defecation an unpleasant side effect of high-fiber diets. Many spend much more time in the toilet.

It would seem more appropriate to strike a middle course. On the Natural Diet there is a natural increase in fiber intake, especially when the diet includes such grains as bran. Until the benefits of high-fiber diets are documented, the wholesale addition of unrefined bran or fiber to the diet seems premature. Because of its nature, the Natural Diet will supply a much more moderate increase in natural fiber without special supplements. For those with special problems such as constipation, special solutions may be appropriate, but most people do not have special problems.

These are a few of the facts about fiber that you should know. Many of the extravagant claims you read in magazines and books are just that—extravagant claims. Remember that most of the current proponents of fiber diets have researched their cures just about as well as the snake-oil merchants researched theirs. If you try an untested diet, *you* are the laboratory animal.

15.

Reviewing the Natural Diet

The fool that eats till he is sick must fast till he is well.
—Walter Thornbury

Even today in certain areas of the world, some people live in constant fear of famine. In the past, in order to survive, most people had to struggle for enough food. Today, most of us live to eat. It is easy to gain weight and frustratingly difficult to lose it. Slimness is the latest fashion, so now we struggle to eat less for our health and appearance.

The family kitchen table is the source of our present eating patterns. But have you ever thought of these patterns as habits? As children we learned to eat what our parents liked. We learned to clean our plates, we learned lollipops made scraped knees feel better, and milk and cookies often soothed a child's hurt. Most of us continue this pattern, eating basically the same foods, in the same amounts and at about the same time every day. In return for a diet which is rich, varied, delightful, and tasteful, we are on the verge of a new problem—overnutrition, particularly overconsumption of certain types of food. Just as we can eat ourselves into obesity and a high risk of heart attack, we can also eat our way out of these dangers. Most important, the change required is simple—not a drastic surrendering of all the foods which tempt you. All you need to do is make a change in the type and amount of *fat* you eat. Since vegetable fats can be tastily and attractively substituted for animal fats in your meal pattern, chances are that you won't even miss your old eating habits. It gets easier as these new patterns replace your old habits, and you begin to enjoy your new eating style.

In an attempt to help yourself, follow these suggestions:

1. Eat a balanced diet as outlined in the diet plan. You will find yourself losing weight while avoiding monotonous restrictions of fad diets.

2. Use low-fat animal products such as skim milk, margarine, egg whites, and low-fat cottage cheese. Not only are these low in calories, but you will also be eliminating much of the cholesterol which is part of the usual affluent diet.

3. Increase your weekly intake of poultry and fish (the amount specified in the diet plan), while limiting your beef intake to twenty ounces a week.

4. Eat slowly and learn to stop eating before you feel full, even if you have not cleaned your plate.

5. Do not skip meals; it is easier to overeat if you are overhungry.

6. Avoid refined sugar and other concentrated sweets such as syrups, jams, jellies, and candy. Also avoid baked goods: cakes, pastries, cookies, etc. These foods provide many calories in a relatively small bulk.

7. When you feel hungry during the day, try some foods which contain negligible calories. These include raw vegetables, diet soda, diet gelatin, broth, and coffee and tea without cream and sugar.

8. Watch the size of your portions. If you cheat, you only cheat yourself!

This is a time of adventure; try new foods, new cooking methods, new recipes. After you decide what changes you are going to make, adopt a positive attitude toward the changes and reward yourself for success. Buy a new dress, a body shirt, or go out and do something new.

The meal plans presented here are kept simple for your ease in using them. Remember that some modification, such as an extra ounce of meat or one serving less of cereal, is not critical or fatal; but eventually you must settle on a plan similar to the one outlined. Permit it to guide you, check yourself by using a diet diary, and then settle down and relax. The weight will come off, and you'll be pleased. Don't expect weight losses that are fantastic, sudden, and unrealistic; remember that fantasy belongs in science fiction, not in a book to reeducate you about your use of food.

The table opposite represents an analysis of the Natural Diet's nutritional components. Remember that you don't have to count calories on this diet, since it is done for you by using the exchange or equivalent system. Remember to adhere as closely as possible to the various quantities that constitute a serving. The table shows the carbohydrate, protein, fat, and caloric analysis of the food groups, as well as a listing of the total servings for the day. Note that there is a range of five to seven servings of bread or cereal and five to six servings of meat. If you use the highest range for one, you should use the lower range of the other. Plan on eleven to twelve servings per day. Remember that the serving size is approximately an ounce.

The table on page 132 provides a nutritional analysis of similar Natural Diet meals, with slightly different amounts of cereal and meat servings in each.

FOOD GROUP ANALYSIS

Meal	Food Group	Servings	Carbo-hydrate (grams)	Protein (grams)	Fat (grams)	Calories
Breakfast	Fruit	1	10			40
	Milk (skim or low-fat)	1 cup	12	8		80
	Bread	1	15	2		68
	Meat	1		7	5	73
	Fat	1			5	45
Lunch	Fruit	1	10			40
	Bread	2	30	4		136
	Vegetable	1				0
	Meat	2		14	10	146
	Fat	1			5	45
Dinner	Fruit	1	10			40
	Bread	1	15	2		68
	Vegetable	1				0
	Meat	3		21	15	219
	Fat	1			5	45
Snack	Milk (skim or low-fat)	1 cup	12	8		80
	Bread	1	15	2		68
Daily Total	2 cups low-fat or skim milk 3 servings fruit 5–7 servings bread 5–6 servings meat 3 servings fat 2 servings vegetables		129 (43.2%)	68 (22.8%)	45 (34%)	1,193

The recommended daily allowances (RDAs) for both men and women are listed on top, men above women. Values are calculated for calcium, iron, vitamins A and C, thiamin, riboflavin, and niacin. Note that either format of the Natural Diet supplies adequate amounts of these nutrients for both men and women. Our studies have demonstrated that people who follow the Natural Diet do not feel hungry or deprived. The simple truth is that they are being adequately nourished while on the diet. That is the secret of why they felt so well—and so will you.

NUTRITIONAL ANALYSIS OF SIMILAR MEALS

Recommended Daily Allowance (Men/Women)	800 mg. Calcium	10 (men) 10–18 mg. (women) Iron	4,000 5,000 IU Vitamin A	45 mg. Vitamin C	1.2–1.4 1.0 mg. Thiamin	1.5–1.6 1.1–1.2 mg. Riboflavin	16–18 12–13 mg. Niacin
2 cups milk	576.0	0.2	700	4.0	0.16	0.84	0.2
3 fruits (1 citrus)	44.0	1.35	630	68.0	0.15	0.11	1.16
5 breads (1 cereal, 1 potato)	185.7	6.6	trace	20.0	0.76	0.51	7.1
6 meats	10.0	2.4	10	—	0.09	0.21	4.7
3 fats	3.0	—	510	—	—	—	—
2 vegetables	51.7	1.53	3,241	31.5	0.166	0.14	1.9
Total	870.4	12.08	5,091	123.5	1.326	1.81	15.06
2 cups milk	576.0	0.2	700	4.0	0.16	0.84	0.2
3 fruits (1 citrus)	44.0	1.35	630	68.0	0.15	0.11	1.16
7 breads (1 cereal, 1 potato)	302.2	10.2	trace	20.0	1.12	0.81	10.7
5 meats	16.0	4.0	16	—	0.15	0.35	7.7
2 fats	1.0	—	340	—	—	—	—
2 vegetables	51.7	1.53	3,241	31.5	0.166	0.14	1.9
Total	990.9	17.28	4,927	123.5	1.746	2.25	21.66

16.

History and Mythology of Cereal Grains

Roast with fire, and unleavened bread; and with bitter herbs they shall eat it.

—Exodus

It's time to get off the meat-and-potato diet; the Natural Diet, a nutritionally sound alternative, returns us to some of the values of our ancestors, who lived mainly on cereal grains. The Natural Diet is an old approach to a new disease, since coronary artery disease and obesity are diseases of the affluent. It is also a successful, painless method of achieving and then maintaining ideal weight, which is indispensable for good health. It seems appropriate here to discuss the history of grains and how they evolved to become a diet staple.

At the end of the Ice Age, a hybrid form of wheat suddenly evolved from wild grasses. This wheat, whose seed was too heavy to be wind-borne, necessitated cultivation. The happy combination of wheat and people created the miracle of agriculture; both became rooted in the soil as, despite the vagaries of temperature and rainfall, purposeful cultivation was obviously more productive and better able to feed a large, growing population than nomadic hunting and gathering had been. Tribes that had previously remained in one place only long enough to exhaust the available food supplies began, with cultivation, to settle in circumscribed areas.

People developed specialized services and skills necessary to survive by communal living. Population density increased as more and more productive and manageable grains evolved. More land meant more food, more power, and more wealth.

Cereals have been important as food since prehistoric times. Included in ancient Greek mythology is a charming story about the grain harvest. Ceres, an agricultural deity from whose name the word *cereal* was derived, was a sister of Zeus, and had an incestuous affair with him. (That was par for many early Greek gods.) The offspring of this tryst was a daughter, Persephone, who came to be called the "grain girl." As she roamed the wheat fields one day, the earth opened up and her Uncle Hades, god of the Underworld, appeared, seized her, and took her to his palace in the Underworld. There she was raped. When Ceres discovered her daughter missing, she withheld her help from the wheat and no more grain grew.

After a year of famine, Zeus decided a compromise must be reached. He convinced his brother Hades to release Persephone if she did not eat while she was in the Underworld. Hades offered Persephone a pomegranate from which she ate only a few seeds, but this meant that she could not freely return to earth. Eventually, she was allowed to return to her mother, Ceres, for part of the year, but was required to return to Hades as queen of the Underworld for three or four months a year. So the myth explains the growing seasons, the birth of the plants in the spring, and their inexorable death after harvest. It was fanciful, but it made sense to those ancient people.

As cereal is more abundant now, so too are meat, milk, eggs, cheese, ice cream, pizza, chocolate, cake, and french fries. Two thoughts suggest themselves: (1) people are eating themselves to death; and (2) it may be that people can and should live on bread alone.

As you read in Chapter 11, there is a direct link between cholesterol and your personal risk of developing heart disease. No responsible authority denies it. The quibbling is over the ability of change in cholesterol intake to effect change of risk status. You can decide for yourself whether to act on the available information. Remember, inaction will let nature take its course, and the natural history of atherosclerotic disease is relentless progression. While the academicians ponder, people with high cholesterol are progressively narrowing their arteries.

The Natural Diet is a responsible approach to the solution of the Erisichthon syndrome. (Erisichthon was a king in ancient Greece who was afflicted with insatiable hunger and, after a series of failing stratagems, was forced to devour himself.) It will provide a livable alternative to the way people are harming themselves nutritionally. Eating cereals can become a way of extending your life rather than merely providing for daily sustenance. The lowered daily intake of cholesterol, calories, and fats afforded by the Natural Diet does make a difference—it is not mythical.

There are unsatisfactory alternatives to following the Natural Diet. Many people take a variety of drugs, such as Atromid S and Questran, to lower their serum lipids. Each of these drugs has the potential of serious side effects. Each is expensive and inconvenient to take. None will lower lipids for everyone.

The Natural Diet has no significant side effects. Instead of costing you money, the Natural Diet will save you money. It has proven to be especially effective in people with high initial levels of cholesterol and triglycerides.

It is the way to go. It will help you become thinner and will reduce your personal risk of suffering the most common disabling diseases of our affluent age. It is truly the staff of life for those who abide by it. It is an idea whose time has come—again.

17.

The Erisichthon Syndrome

Kill not your hearts with excess eating and drinking.

—Mohammed

Chameleons feed on light and air,
Poets' food is love and fame.

—Percy Bysshe Shelley

Unlike Shelley's chameleons and poets, the rest of us require food. Food contains calories, protein, carbohydrates, fats, vitamins, minerals, and several trace elements. Denied food, we die. How well and how long we live are determined very much by how well we eat. Food has wonderful power that permits us to work, grow, and reproduce. It helps the body repair itself, and protects us from disease. But food does not have magical properties. It cannot bring happiness, nor can it be consumed endlessly without harming the body.

The Talmud said: "More people die from overeating than from undernourishment." The dangers of overeating have now been documented to include an increased incidence of hypertension (high blood pressure), diabetes mellitus, and excessive accumulation of fatty materials in the blood. (Some of these increase the risk of heart attack and stroke.)

Despite the ready availability of adequate and varied food supplies, Americans do not uniformly enjoy good nutrition. Many more people suffer from excessive food intake than from starvation. Even the ancients were aware of the importance of eating and the dangers of stuffing oneself. Theognis wrote in 600 B.C, "Surfeit has killed many more men than famine." The Greeks believed in moderation in all things. Certain biblical writings label gluttony a sin.

In a very literal way many modern Americans are eating themselves to death, just as Erisichthon did. Like many myths, the story of Erisichthon is undoubtedly based on the experience of ancient people. They were keen

141

observers and recognized that the more gluttonous members of their society tended to die earlier and of more sudden, catastrophic diseases.

We have Erisichthons in our midst, armies of people killing themselves with their mouths. They eat too much and move too little. The Erisichthons of today are busily eating high-fat, high-cholesterol, calorie-laden food. They accumulate pounds and inches, growing ever closer to degenerative and vascular disease. The problem is their eating habits. Unable to deny themselves instant gratification in order to reach long-range goals, they make no attempt to modify their behavior.

Like Erisichthon, they are self-destructive; they disregard whatever knowledge they have about good nutrition and health. Sometimes ignorance is the excuse; more often it is unwillingness to come to grips with reality. No one can eat everything without eventually paying the price in terms of health, ability, and well-being. In the affluent West, people eat vast quantities of food without regard to balanced nutrition or the long-range effect on their bodies. Much of what we crave is learned—dictated by massive and persuasive advertising.

The Erisichthon syndrome is a creation of our own making. Like all such problems, it is reversible, and enlightened self-interest is the most powerful tool to effect this reversal. Only if we understand what constitutes good nutrition can we hope to relegate the Erisichthon syndrome to the category of a rare medical oddity. At present it is an illness of epidemic proportions.

Recipes

The following recipes demonstrate the wide variety of delicious foods which the ideal diet permits. Many of these recipes were contributed by the volunteers who followed the diet themselves. For convenience, the recipes are arranged in four main groups of soups, salads, main dishes, and desserts, breads, and snacks. Preceding each recipe you will find the exchange value for one serving. The number of servings is given after the recipe. I must emphasize that in addition to following the recipes you should try some of your own favorite foods, modified to contain lower amounts of fat, calories, and cholesterol. You should learn to use diet margarine in food preparation, as well as diet salad dressing and low-sugar desserts.

SOUPS

AUNT LUCY'S CARROT SOUP
(1 bread)

1 large onion, sliced	3 ¼ cup sliced carrots
2 Tbs. margarine	1 cup minced celery
1 Tbs. flour	2 tsp. salt
4 cups beef broth	½ tsp. pepper

Brown the onion in melted margarine, stir in flour, and add beef broth. Keep stirring until mixture begins to boil. Cook 3 minutes. Add carrots, celery, salt, and pepper and let simmer 1 hour. Put through a food mill or sieve and serve hot. Serves 6.

COUNTRY GARDEN SOUP
(1 bread)

1 carrot, diced	1 leek, sliced
½ small turnip, diced	½ cup shelled peas
½ cup shredded cabbage	½ potato, diced
1 Tbs. margarine	1 tsp. minced parsley
3 cups beef broth	Salt and pepper to taste

Sauté carrot, turnip, and cabbage in margarine. Add broth, leek, peas, potato, parsley, and salt and pepper. Cover and simmer for 1 hour. Serves 4.

AUNT SADIE'S SPINACH BORSCHT
(1 oz. meat, 1 fat)

1 lb. spinach, washed and chopped	Salt and sugar to taste
1 lb. rhubarb, cut in small pieces	2 low-cholesterol eggs
6 cups water	Imitation diet sour cream

Boil spinach, rhubarb, water, and seasonings together until rhubarb has dissolved. Beat eggs and slowly add borscht. Chill and serve with imitation sour cream. Serves 6.

MAMA'S CHICKEN SOUP
(1 bread, 4 chicken)

1 3–4-lb. chicken, cut in pieces	2 stalks celery and celery tips
3 ½ qts. water	8 peppercorns
1 large onion	1 tsp. dill weed
3 carrots	Salt and pepper to taste

Place chicken in pot with water, cover tightly, and let simmer 3 hours or until chicken has begun to be tender. Add vegetables and seasonings and let simmer another hour. Strain and remove fat. Serves 6.

TOMATO-CABBAGE SOUP
(1 bread, 2 meat)

¾ lb. chuck beef	2 apples
1 marrow bone	2 cups strained tomatoes
1 ½ qts. cold water	Salt and pepper to taste
1 medium cabbage head	

Place meat and bone in soup pot with cold water, heat to boiling point and let simmer 45 minutes. Shred and add cabbage; slice and add apples and tomatoes. Let simmer 30 minutes or until meat and cabbage are tender. Add salt and pepper, let boil gently 1 minute, and serve. Serves 6.

MINESTRONE SOUP
(1 bread)

1 cup green or yellow split peas
1 carrot, diced
1 onion; whole
2 qts. water

1 soupbone
1 can vegetarian vegetable soup
Salt and pepper to taste

Boil vegetables and soupbone in water until peas are tender. Add soup, salt and pepper, and simmer for about 1 hour. Serves 6.

VEGETABLE SOUP
(1 bread)

2 cups dried lima beans
1 large soupbone
2 cups tomatoes
2 cups grated corn
2 cups chopped cabbage
1 large turnip, diced

1 carrot, diced
1 onion, sliced
Salt and pepper to taste
1 tsp. flour
½ cup skim milk
3 quarts water

Soak lima beans in cold water for several hours. Meanwhile, wash soupbone, cover with cold water, and boil slowly for several hours. Skim off fat from top, add vegetables and drained beans. Season to taste. Cook until vegetables are tender, 1 hour. Mix flour with milk and stir into soup. Cook 15 minutes and serve hot. Serves 10.

OKRA SOUP
(1 bread)

1 soupbone
4 cups cold water
4 cups sliced okra

2 cups skinned tomatoes
Salt and pepper to taste

Cover soupbone with cold water and heat to boiling; cook about 1 hour. Add okra, tomatoes, and seasoning. Simmer for 2 hours or until thick. Serve with rice or noodles. Serves 6.

POTATO-LEEK SOUP
(1 bread, 1 fat)

4 cups diced potatoes
4 cups sliced leeks
6 cups chicken broth
½ cup skim milk

2 Tbs. safflower oil
1 tsp. salt
Pepper to taste
Minced parsley

Simmer potatoes and leeks in chicken broth until tender. Add milk, oil, salt, and pepper. Simmer 30 minutes. Garnish with parsley and serve. Serves 8.

BOUILLABAISE A LA GREQUE
(1 bread, 2 meat, 1 fat)

3—4 lbs. mixed fresh fish
   (including seafood)
10 cups water
1 lb. sliced onions
1 lb. tomatoes, peeled and sliced

⅓ cup safflower oil
2 Tbs. olive oil
1 tsp. salt
½ tsp. pepper

Clean and wash fish. Put remaining ingredients in a large soup pot and bring to a boil. Add smaller fish and let simmer for 1½ hours. Add larger fish, including lobster and shrimp, and simmer 20 minutes. Remove larger fish and put soup through a food mill to make a thick stock. Transfer stock to tureen and add larger fish. Serves 10.

GREEK RICE SOUP
(1 bread, 1 meat)

12 cups chicken broth
12 Tbs. uncooked long-grain rice
Pinch of salt

12 Tbs. egg substitute
Juice of 2 lemons

Bring chicken broth to a boil, add rice and salt, and cook over low heat until rice is tender. Beat egg substitute and lemon juice in bowl. Gradually add 1 cup of the stock by spoonfuls, stirring constantly. Pour egg-lemon mixture into remaining stock in soup pot. Heat over very low heat, stirring constantly. Do not let mixture boil. Serve immediately. Serves 8.

TOMATO AND PASTA SOUP
(1 bread, 1 fat)

1 lb. ripe tomatoes, sliced
1 carrot, sliced
1 stalk celery
6 cups chicken broth
½ cup safflower oil

1 tsp. olive oil
Salt and pepper to taste
1 cup vermicelli
Chopped parsley

Put all ingredients except vermicelli into a pan and cook slowly for ½ hour. Force through a sieve and bring again to a boil. Add vermicelli and continue cooking for about 10 minutes. Add parsley. Serves 6.

SALADS

VEGETABLE SKILLET SALAD
(1 bread)

2 medium onions, thinly sliced
2 Tbs. margarine
1 3-oz. can (⅔ cup) sliced mushrooms
4 medium zucchini, thinly sliced
   (5—6 cups)

1 tsp. salt
Dash of pepper
2 tomatoes, cut in 16 wedges

In skillet, cook onions in margarine until tender-crisp. Drain mushrooms, reserving 2 Tbs. liquid. Add zucchini, mushrooms, mushroom liquid, salt, and pepper to skillet. Cook, covered, until squash is tender, about 8 minutes. Add tomatoes. Heat through. Serves 4–6.

CUSTARD SPINACH
(½ milk, 1 egg, 1 fat)

½ cup cooked, chopped spinach   ⅓ cup egg substitute
½ cup skim milk   1 tsp. margarine
Salt and pepper to taste

Preheat oven to 350°. Mix spinach, milk, and salt and pepper together. Beat egg substitute and stir the spinach-milk mixture into it. Grease an oven-proof dish with the margarine and pour in custard mixture. Place in a pan of hot water and bake until set, about 30 minutes. Serves 1.

CAULIFLOWER BOWL
(free)

½ cup sliced cauliflower   Salt to taste
½ cup lettuce   Vinegar
½ cup shredded carrots

Slice cauliflower in ¼-in. cuts. Slice the part near the stalk very thin. Tear lettuce. Add carrots and toss. Add salt. Chill. Serve with vinegar. Serves 1.

ORIENTAL SALAD
(free)

¼ cup chopped spinach   ¼ cup thinly sliced green pepper
¼ cup torn lettuce   ¼ cup shredded cabbage
¼ cup drained bean sprouts   ¼ cup watercress
¼ cup sliced celery   2 Tbs. soy sauce
⅛ cup water chestnuts   Vinegar to taste
¼ cup mushrooms

Combine all vegetables. Blend in soy sauce. Add vinegar. Toss. Serves 1.

SUMMER SALAD
(1 oz. meat)

1 pkg. unsweetened lime gelatin   1 tsp. chopped green pepper
1 cup hot water   ½ cup shredded carrots
1 tsp. lemon juice   ¼ cup cottage cheese
½ tsp. grated onion   Lettuce leaves
Salt and pepper to taste

Dissolve gelatin in hot water. Add lemon juice, onion, and salt and pepper. Add green pepper, carrots, and cottage cheese. Blend well. Chill in mold. When firm, remove from mold. Serve on lettuce leaves. Serves 4.

FRUITED CABBAGE
(1 fruit, 1 oz. meat)

½ cup shredded cabbage
½ cup unsweetened canned
  fruit cocktail, drained
¼ cup cottage cheese

1 Tbs. lemon juice
Salt and pepper to taste
Lettuce leaf

Toss cabbage and fruit together. Mix in cottage cheese. Add lemon juice, salt, and pepper. Chill. Serve on lettuce leaf. Serves 1.

POTATO SALAD
(1 bread, 1 fat)

1 cup diced boiled potato
1 ½ tsp. chopped pimento
¼ cup diced celery
1 ½ tsp. chopped onion
1 Tbs. chopped parsley
1 tsp. vinegar

½ tsp. dry mustard
½ tsp. celery seed
Dash of pepper
¼ tsp. salt
1 ½ Tbs. mayonnaise

Combine all ingredients except mayonnaise and lettuce. Chill. Before serving, add mayonnaise. Serve on lettuce leaf. Serves 2.

GARDEN MOLD
(free)

1 pkg. unflavored gelatin
1 ¾ cups broth or bouillon
2 Tbs. unsweetened lemon juice
¼ tsp. salt
½ cup chopped spinach

6 cucumber slices, halved
½ cup chopped celery
¼ cup sliced radishes
½ cup chopped carrots

Sprinkle gelatin over ¾ cup of broth in a saucepan. Heat slowly until dissolved. Remove from heat. Add remaining broth, lemon juice, and salt. Chill until slightly thickened. Stir in vegetables. Pour into mold. Chill. Serves 4.

TOMATO ASPIC SALAD
(free)

1 ¾ cups tomato juice
½ tsp. salt
⅛ tsp. pepper
1 bay leaf
½ tsp. paprika
1 tsp. unsweetened lemon juice

1 Tbs. chopped onion
1 pkg. unflavored gelatin
¼ cup cold water
½ cup chopped celery
2 Tbs. chopped parsley
¼ cup chopped green pepper

Heat tomato juice, salt, pepper, and bay leaf. Take out bay leaf. Add paprika, lemon juice, and onion. Soften gelatin in cold water. Combine with tomato-juice mixture and stir until dissolved. Cool. Add chopped vegetables. Refrigerate until firm. Serves 2.

THREE BEAN SALAD
(1 fat, 2 bread)

1 can green beans	¾ cup sugar substitute
1 can yellow wax beans	⅔ cup vinegar
1 can kidney beans	⅓ cup vegetable oil
1 can chick-peas	1 tsp. salt
1 green pepper, sliced	¼ tsp. pepper
1 onion, sliced	

Drain beans and chick-peas. Add green pepper and onion. Make dressing of remaining ingredients and add. Let stand overnight. Serves 8.

GELATIN SALAD
(2 meat, 1 fruit, 1 fat)

1 3-oz. pkg. lemon or lime diet gelatin	1 can mandarin oranges, drained
1 lb. skim-milk cottage cheese	1 pt. diet whip cream substitute
1 can crushed pineapple packed in its own juice, drained	

Stir dry gelatin into cottage cheese. Add pineapple, oranges, and whip. Chill until set. Serves 6.

JELLIED CRANBERRY SALAD
(1 fruit)

2 cups cranberries	1 cup sugar substitute
1 apple, peeled	1 3-oz. package lemon diet gelatin
Skin from 1 lemon and 1 orange	1 cup boiling water

Grind fruits and skins, add sweetener, and let stand 1 hour. Mix gelatin with water. Add to fruit mixture, pour into mold, and chill until firm. Serves 4.

ANTIPASTO I
(1 fruit, 2 meat, 1 fat)

2 7-oz. tins tuna, packed in water	1 bottle chili sauce
1 jar small gherkins, sliced	1 bottle catsup
1 can button mushrooms	1 Tbs. Worcestershire sauce
1 can chopped green olives	Juice of 1 lemon
1 jar pickled cauliflower	1 bottle white horseradish
1 jar pickled onions	

Drain tuna and vegetables. Add seasonings as desired (use horseradish to taste) and mix. Serves 4.

ANTIPASTO II
(4 meat, 1 bread)

½ cup tuna fish, drained
1 oz. low-cholesterol cheese, cut in cubes
½ cup cooked rice
½ cup small mushrooms

8 pickled onions
1 green pepper, diced
2 tomatoes, sliced
Salt and pepper to taste

Mix all ingredients together. Serves 1.

SALADE NICOISE
(3 meat, 3 fat, 3 bread)

2 tsp. Dijon mustard
⅓ cup vinegar
1 ½ tsp. salt
1 or 2 cloves garlic, finely minced
10 Tbs. safflower oil
1 Tbs. olive oil
Freshly ground black pepper to taste
1 tsp. chopped fresh or ½ tsp. dried thyme
1 ½ lbs. fresh green beans
2 green peppers
4 ribs celery

1 pt. cherry tomatoes
5 medium-sized red-skinned potatoes, cooked, peeled, and sliced
3 7-oz. cans tuna, packed in water
1 1- or 2-oz. can anchovies
10 stuffed olives
10 black olives
2 small or 1 large red Bermuda onion
2 Tbs. fresh or 1 tsp. dried basil
½ cup finely chopped fresh parsley
¼ cup finely chopped green onions

In a mixing bowl, combine mustard, vinegar, salt garlic, oils, pepper, and thyme. Beat with a fork until well blended. Set dressing aside.

Pick over beans and break into 1 ½-inch lengths. Place in a saucepan and cook in salted water to cover until tender but crisp. Drain and run under cold water. Remove cores from green peppers. Remove seeds and white membranes. Cut peppers into thin rounds. Set aside. Trim celery ribs. Cut crosswise into thin slices. There should be about 2 cups of sliced celery.

Use a large salad bowl and make a symmetrical pattern of the green beans, peppers, celery, tomatoes, and potatoes. Flake tuna fish and add to bowl. Arrange anchovies on top and scatter olives over all. Peel onions and cut into thin, almost transparent slices. Scatter onion rings over all. Sprinkle with basil, parsley, and green onions.

Toss salad with dressing after garnished bowl has been presented to guests for their enjoyment. Serve with crusty French or Italian bread. Serves 6.

ORANGE-ARTICHOKE SALAD
(1 fruit, 1 bread, 1 fat)

1 can artichoke hearts, drained	Dash of oregano
Naval orange segments to equal 1 can	Salt to taste
2 Tbs. orange juice	Lettuce
2 cloves garlic, minced	

Mix ingredients and serve on bed of crisp lettuce. Serves 4.

WHITE BEAN SALAD
(1 fat, 4 bread)

1 lb. white beans	Parsley, dill, or mint
2 tsp. salt	Dried or fresh spring onions
½ cup diet Italian dressing	

Soak beans overnight. Drain; cover with cold water and boil 1 ½ hours. Add salt and continue to cook for ½ hour or until beans are tender. Cool and drain. Mix beans with dressing. Chop herbs and onion and sprinkle over beans. Serves 3.

LIME-CUCUMBER RING
(2 fruit)

2 packages diet lime gelatin	1 tsp. salt
3 ¾ cups boiling water	1 can crushed pineapple, 20 oz.,
Juice of 1 lemon	packed in its own juice
¼ cup vinegar	2 carrots, grated
½ cup sugar	1 cucumber, grated

Dissolve gelatin in hot water. Add rest of ingredients. Put small amount of clear liquid in mold. When partially set, add rest of mixture and fill ring mold. Let set. Serves 6.

LOW-CALORIE COTTAGE CHEESE SALAD
(2 oz. meat)

2 cups skim-milk cottage cheese	6 scallions, chopped very fine
10 radishes, sliced very thin	Salt and pepper to taste
2 small cucumbers, sliced thin	

Combine cottage cheese and vegetables. Add salt and pepper. Serves 4.

CONNIE'S MUSHROOM SURPRISE
(free)

1 medium onion	1 can stewed tomatoes
1 Tbs. safflower oil	Seasoning to taste
5 cups mushrooms	

Sauté onion in oil. Add mushrooms, tomatoes and seasoning. Simmer for 20 minutes. Serves 12.

VINAIGRETTE DRESSING
(1 Tbs. = 1 fat)

½ cup corn oil
2 Tbs. wine vinegar
1 tsp. oregano
½ tsp. salt

¼ tsp. pepper
¼ tsp. dry mustard
1 crushed garlic clove

Combine ingredients. Shake. Serve on tossed salad.

TOMATO DRESSING
(free)

½ cup tomato juice
2 Tbs. vinegar
1 Tbs. chopped onion

Salt and pepper to taste
½ tsp. chopped parsley

Combine ingredients. Shake. Serve on green salad.

LEMON DRESSING
(free)

1 lemon
1 small clove garlic, crushed

1 ½ tsp. corn oil

Squeeze juice from lemon and mix with garlic and oil. Let stand for 2 or more hours. Remove garlic. Serve on salad greens, sparingly.

MAIN DISHES

HAMBURGER STROGANOFF
(2 bread, 1 fat, 2 oz. meat)

1 lb. lean ground beef
1 medium onion
1 can mushrooms
1 can mushroom soup

1 small container low-calorie sour
   cream
1 bag noodles or rice (4 cups cooked)

Brown meat in Teflon pan (no oil). Chop onion and add to meat. Add mushrooms and soup. Simmer for 20 minutes. Add sour cream and heat through. Pour over noodles or rice. Serves 6.

BROWNED RICE
(1 bread, 1 fat)

1 medium onion, chopped
¼ lb. margarine
1 cup rice, uncooked

1 can mushrooms
1 can consomme
1 cup water

Preheat oven to 350°. Sauté onion in margarine in heavy skillet. Remove onion and set aside. Add rice to margarine and brown very slowly, stirring constantly. When rice is cooked, mix with onion, mushrooms, and liquids. Bake in

9 x 13-inch uncovered casserole in oven until liquid is absorbed. Stir occasionally while rice cooks. Serves 4.

BULGHUR WHEAT
(1 bread)

1 cup bulghur wheat	½ tsp. salt
2 Tbs. sliced green onion	¼ tsp. thyme
2 Tbs. margarine	⅛ tsp. cumin
2 cups chicken broth	

Sauté wheat and green onions in margarine until golden. Add broth and spices. Cover and bring to boil. Turn off heat and leave on burner until soft. Serves 4.

TABBOULEH
(1 bread, 1 fat)

1 cup fine bulghur wheat	¼ tsp. freshly ground black pepper
¾ cup onion, chopped	1 ½ cups finely chopped Italian parsley
½ cup scallions with green parts finely chopped	1 tsp. olive oil
1 tsp. salt	2 tomatoes skinned and cut into wedges

Cover bulghur wheat with cold water and let stand 1 hour. Drain and squeeze out extra water. Add the remaining ingredients except the tomatoes and mix well with the hands. Pile into a dish and garnish with the tomatoes. Serves 6.

HELENE'S SPANISH RICE
(2 meat, 2 bread)

1 lb. lean ground beef	4 cups cooked rice
1 can stewed tomatoes	Seasoning to taste
3 Tbs. tomato paste	

Brown meat in a Teflon pan (no oil or fat). Add rice, tomatoes, tomato paste, and seasoning and cook for 20 minutes over medium heat. Serves 4-6.

SPAGHETTI
(1 fat, 2 meat, 1 bread)

1 Tbs. chopped onion	Salt and pepper to taste
2 oz. beef, ground	¼ cup water
1 Tbs. oil	½ cup spaghetti, cooked
½ cup cooked tomato	1 tsp. grated Italian cheese
2 Tbs. tomato paste	

Brown onion and meat in oil. Add tomato, tomato paste, salt and pepper, and water. Simmer for 1 to 2 hours. If necessary, add more water. Serve over spaghetti and sprinkle with cheese. Serves 1.

MILAN-STYLE RICE
(2 fat, 1 bread, 1 meat)

1 slice onion
2 tsp. diet margarine
½ cup cooked rice
1 cup hot water

Salt to taste
1 thread saffron
¼ cup broth or bouillon
1 oz. Parmesan cheese

Brown onion in 1 tsp. margarine. Add rice and stir. Pour in hot water and continue to stir. Add salt. When cooked dry, add 1 tsp. margarine. Dissolve saffron in warm broth and add rice until yellow. Sprinkle with cheese. Serves 1.

FOIL DINNER
(3 oz. meat)

3 oz. lean ground beef
1 tsp. cholesterol-free egg
Mixed vegetable juice
Salt and pepper to taste

1 carrot
1 stalk celery
1 small onion

Preheat oven to 375°. Mix beef with egg and enough juice to moisten well. Add salt and pepper. Place on sheet of aluminum foil. Slice carrot and celery and dice onion. Place vegetable on top of beef. Fold foil to seal. Bake in oven for 35 minutes. If no bread is being used for meal, 1 small potato may be sliced in with the vegetables. Serves 1.

FARMER'S EGGPLANT
(3 oz. meat, 1 fat, 2 bread)

2 medium eggplants
1 large onion, sliced
2 tsp. diet margarine
1 lb. ground beef

1 cup bread crumbs
Salt and pepper to taste
6 Tbs. egg substitute
Grated cheese

Preheat oven to 400°. Boil eggplants until soft. Split them open, remove the pulp, put in a flat pan, and mash. Set aside. Fry onion in 1 tsp. margarine until soft. Add beef and cook 5 minutes; add to eggplant with bread crumbs and salt and pepper. Add egg substitute and mix well. Butter a casserole with remaining margarine, put in eggplant mixture, and sprinkle the top with grated cheese. Bake in oven for 35 to 40 minutes. Serves 6.

CABBAGE AND BEEF CASSEROLE
(3 oz. meat, 1 bread, 1 fat)

1 medium onion
3 tsp. diet margarine
½ lb. ground beef
½ tsp. salt

¼ tsp pepper
6 cups coarsely shredded cabbage
1 10½-oz. can tomato soup

Preheat oven to 350°. Sauté onion in 2 teaspoons margarine. Add the ground beef, salt, and pepper. Heat through but do not brown. Spread 3 cups of the cabbage in a casserole greased with remaining margarine. Cover with the meat mixture, and place the rest of the cabbage on top. Pour tomato soup over all. Bake 1 hour in oven. Serves 2.

EASY OVEN CASSEROLE
(2 bread, 3 meat)

2 cups raw diced potatoes
2 cups chopped celery
2 cups ground beef
1 cup finely chopped green pepper

2 cans canned tomatoes
1 cup sliced onions
Salt and pepper to taste

Preheat oven to 375°. Place ingredients in baking dish in order given. Sprinkle with salt and pepper. Bake in oven for 1 ½ hours. Serves 6.

ITALIAN-STYLE BEEF
(3 oz. meat, 1 bread, 1 fat)

1 garlic clove, minced
1 tsp. corn oil
⅓ cup canned tomatoes
Dash of oregano

Salt and pepper to taste
3 oz. diced beef
Chopped parsley
½ cup spaghetti, cooked

Brown garlic in oil. Add tomatoes, oregano, and salt and pepper and cook at low heat for 15 minutes. Add meat and cook another 15 minutes. Sprinkle with parsley. Serve with spaghetti. Serves 1.

PORK CHOP CASSEROLE
(3 oz. meat, 1 bread)

1 3-oz. pork chop, trimmed
½ cup noodles
1 tsp. onion salt

Salt and pepper to taste
Pinch of sage
½ cup tomato juice

Preheat oven to 350°. Brown pork chop on both sides in Teflon pan. Cook noodles and place in a small oven-proof dish. Add seasonings to tomato juice. Pour over noodles. Place pork chop on noodles. Cover and bake for ½ hour. Serves 1.

HAM HAWAIIAN
(½ milk, 3 oz. meat, 1 fruit)

3-oz. lean ham slice
1 unsweetened pineapple ring
3 Tbs. unsweetened pineapple juice
8 cloves

1 small apple
½ cup skim milk
Chopped parsley

Preheat oven to 350°. Place ham in oven-proof frying pan. Place pineapple on ham and pour juice over it. Place cloves around pineapple. With a melon scoop, cut out 1 ball of the apple and place in center of pineapple ring. Pour milk over ham and bake in oven for ¾ hour. Garnish with parsley and serve. Serves 1.

CABBAGE DELIGHT
(3 oz. meat)

3 oz. ground beef, cooked
1 Tbs. chopped onion
1 tsp. diced green pepper

Salt and pepper to taste
1 large cabbage leaf
½ cup tomato juice

Preheat oven to 375°. Lightly grease a frying pan and brown meat. Add onion and green pepper and seasoning. Place mixture on cabbage leaf and roll up to cover meat. Put in oven-proof baking dish and pour tomato juice over it. Bake until well cooked. Serves 1.

DUTCH STEAK
(2 oz. meat, 1 fat)

2 oz. round steak
1 ½ tsp. vinegar
Salt and pepper to taste

1 tsp. diet margarine
Water

Tenderize steak by pounding. Put in dish. Rub with vinegar, salt, and pepper, combined as marinade, and allow to stand for ½ hour. Heat margarine in a frying pan, place steak in pan and fry 1 minute on each side while constantly moving steak back and forth in pan. If well-done steak is desired, cook longer. Remove steak to serving dish and add a little water to pan. Allow to boil; serve as gravy. Serves 1.

STEAK WITH TOMATOES AND MUSHROOMS
(3 oz. meat, 1 fat)

3 oz. steak
Salt and pepper to taste
2 tsp. chopped onion

½ cup mushrooms
1 tsp. diet margarine
¾ cup stewed tomatoes

Preheat oven to 300°. Panbroil steak and season with salt and pepper. In an oven-proof pan, brown onions and mushrooms in margarine. Add tomatoes. Pour over steak and return to pan in which fat was melted. Heat in oven for 10 minutes. Serves 1.

STUFFED TOMATO WITH CHICKEN
(1 bread, 1 oz. meat, 1 fat)

1 medium tomato
Salt and pepper
½ cup rice, cooked

1 oz. (¼ cup) ground cooked chicken
1 tsp. diet margarine

Preheat oven to 350°. Cut thin slice off top of tomato and scoop out pulp. Sprinkle inside of tomato with salt and pepper. Mix pulp with the rice and chicken and fill tomato with mixture. Place margarine on tomato and set in lightly oiled pan. Bake for 20 minutes. Serves 1.

HALIBUT CREOLE
(3 oz. meat, 1 fat)

½ cup tomatoes
½ cup water
1 tsp. chopped onion
Salt and pepper to taste

Dash of paprika
1 tsp. diet margarine
3 oz. halibut
Tomato juice (optional)

Preheat oven to 350°. Cook tomatoes, water, onion, salt and pepper, and paprika for 5 minutes. Melt margarine in a frying pan, pour in tomatoes, and brown for another 5 minutes. Place fish in a shallow, greased pan and pour mixture over it. Bake for 15-20 minutes. More water or tomato juice may be added during baking to keep fish moist. Serves 1.

BAKED STUFFED FISH
(3 oz. meat, 1 bread, 1 fat)

6 Fresh brook trout
2 Tbs. lemon juice
1 tsp. salt
2 cups bread crumbs
1 Tbs. grated onion

½ cup chopped celery
2 Tbs. water
Chopped parsley
½ cup chopped mushrooms

Preheat oven to 400°. Slit fish and rub inside with 1 Tbs. lemon juice and ½ tsp. salt. Combine remaining ingredients. Stuff each fish with ⅓ cup bread mixture and fasten edges with skewers. Place on greased foil in shallow baking pan. Brush with oil and bake until done. Do not overcook. Serves 6.

TUNA SPECIAL
(4 oz. meat, 1 fat, ½ milk, 1 bread)

¾ cup sliced mushrooms
2 Tbs. margarine
1 Tbs. flour
1 cup skim milk
½ cup soft bread crumbs

1 7-oz. can tuna, flaked
2 Tbs. chopped parsley
2 Tbs. chopped green pepper
1 tsp. salt
Dash of pepper
⅔ cup egg substitute

Preheat oven to 350°. Sauté mushrooms in margarine. Blend in flour and milk and cook until thickened, stirring continuously. Add bread crumbs, tuna, parsley, green pepper, salt, pepper, and egg substitute. Pour into greased shallow baking dish. Place in shallow pan of hot water and bake for 40 minutes. Serves 2.

FISH STEW
(1 bread, 5 oz. meat)

1 lb. whitefish
1 lb. pike
Juice of ½ lemon
8 cups water
5 potatoes, peeled and cut in
    ¾-in. slices

2 carrots, quartered
4 onions, sliced
1 bay leaf
1 Tbs. salt
⅓ tsp. pepper
Dash of paprika

Wash and slice fish; squeeze lemon juice over fish. Let stand in refrigerator a few hours. Wash slightly and cook in water, adding potatoes, carrots, onions, bay leaf, salt, pepper, and paprika. Simmer 1 hour. Serve very hot. Serves 6.

SALMON LOAF
(½ milk, 4 oz. meat)

1 large can red salmon	1 large onion, grated
6 Tbs. egg substitute	½ cup matzo meal
3 carrots, grated	½ cup cooked green peas
1 cup skim milk	Salt and pepper to taste

Preheat oven to 350°. Drain salmon and flake. Beat egg substitute and add to salmon with remaining ingredients. Place in medium-sized greased loaf pan. Bake for 1 hour. Serves 4.

BROILED WHITEFISH OR HALIBUT
(4 oz. meat, 1 fat, 1 bread)

2 lbs. whitefish or halibut	Paprika
1 cup bread crumbs	3 Tbs. margarine
1 tsp. salt	Juice of ½ lemon
½ tsp. onion salt	1 lemon cut in 6 wedges

Have fish split (if whitefish). Mix bread crumbs with salt, onion salt, and paprika. Melt 2 Tbs. margarine in broiling pan and add lemon juice. Dip each piece of fish in margarine mixture, then roll in seasoned bread crumbs. Place fish, skin side down, on broiling pan. Dot with remaining margarine and broil slowly until well browned, basting with own gravy, about 20 minutes. Serve with lemon wedges. It is not necessary to turn the fish if it is not too thick. Serves 6.

HALIBUT SALAD
(3 oz. meat, 1 fat)

1 lb. halibut	1 hard-boiled egg, cut up
1 tsp. salt	1 tsp. diet mayonnaise
1 onion, peeled and quartered	Salt
2 stalks celery, chopped fine	Lemon juice
1 Tbs. vinegar	Lettuce leaves
½ cup finely chopped celery	

Boil halibut in water to cover. Add salt, onion, celery stalks, vinegar. Boil 20 minutes. Remove fish and when cool, remove skin and bone. Flake fish, add celery, egg, and mayonnaise, salt, and lemon juice to taste. Serve on lettuce. Serves 5 or 6.

PASTA WITH LENTILS
(4 bread)

1 onion, peeled and sliced
2 carrots, diced
2 medium potatoes, peeled and diced
2 tomatoes, peeled and chopped

2 stalks celery, chopped
1 cup dried lentils
Salt and pepper to taste
½ cup Italian pasta, uncooked

Fill a 6-quart pot ⅔ full of water. Add onion, carrots, potatoes, tomatoes, celery, and lentils and simmer for 1 ½ hours. Stir occasionally. Add salt and pepper. During the last 10 minutes of cooking, put in pasta. Cook until pasta is done. Serves 2.

JOE'S PASTA WITH VEGETABLES
(1 fat, 4 bread)

1 medium onion, peeled and sliced
1 Tbs. safflower oil
Salt and pepper to taste
2 Tbs. chopped parsley

1 can chick-peas or white
  navy beans
¾ lb. broken spaghetti or
  small-sized pasta

In a deep frying pan, put enough safflower oil to cover the bottom of the pan. Add onion and sauté until soft. Add salt and pepper and parsley. Simmer 20 minutes to ½ hour. Add peas or beans. In a saucepan, cook pasta in salted water until just barely soft. Drain, keeping some of the water. Mix with vegetable mixture and serve. Serves 4.

VEGETABLE CRISP CASSEROLE
(3 bread, 1 fat)

Spray pan-coater
1 ½ cups carrots, sliced crosswise
1 ½ cups cut green beans
1 ½ cups celery, cut in ½-inch slices
⅔ cup water
¾ tsp. salt
Dash of pepper

½ tsp. thyme
1 Tbs. finely chopped celery leaves
1 Tbs. finely chopped onion
¼ cup diet margarine
1 cup cream of mushroom soup
3 cups bite-size rice biscuits

Preheat oven to 350°. Spray an 8- or 9-inch baking dish with pan-coater. Place carrots, beans, and celery in saucepan with water. Add salt, pepper, and ¼ tsp. thyme. Cover and boil about 15 minutes or until just tender. Strain and reserve liquid. Place vegetables in baking dish. Cook celery leaves and onion in 2 Tbs. margarine until onions are clear. Add soup and ½ cup reserved liquid. Mix well and pour over vegetables. Add 2 Tbs. margarine and remaining thyme to biscuits. Coat and stir over low heat 5 minutes. Crush biscuits slightly and sprinkle over casserole. Bake in oven about 30 minutes or until bubbly and brown. Serves 8.

BUTTERNUT SQUASH
(1 fruit, 2 fat, 1 bread)

1 butternut squash
⅔ cup drained pineapple,
  packed in its own juice

2 Tbs. diet margarine
1 Tbs. lemon juice
Salt and pepper to taste

Cook squash until tender. Remove skin and mash pulp. Add pineapple, margarine, lemon juice, and salt and pepper. Heat and serve. Serves 1.

BAKED PORK CHOPS AND APPLESAUCE
(3 oz. meat, 1 fruit)

6 pork chops
1 large can diet applesauce
¼ tsp. cinnamon

Salt and pepper to taste
½ cup sherry wine

Preheat oven to 350°. Brown chops in heavy skillet. Remove to baking dish. Mix applesauce with cinnamon, salt and pepper, and sherry. Spoon ½ the mixture on chops. Bake 25 minutes in oven. Turn chops and spoon on remainder of applesauce. Return to oven and bake another 25 minutes. Serves 6.

HUNGARIAN VEAL
(3 oz. meat, 1 bread, 1 fat)

1 ½ lb. veal steak, cut in 1-in. pieces
¼ cup flour
1 clove garlic
3 Tbs. margarine
2 Tbs. minced onion

1 Tbs. minced parsley
½ tsp. salt
¼ tsp. paprika
¼ tsp. celery salt
1 cup hot white wine

Roll veal in flour. Brown garlic in melted margarine. Discard the garlic, add onion and veal, and brown together. Add parsley, salt, paprika, celery salt and wine. Simmer 1 hour. Serve with mashed potatoes or rice. Serves 6.

HAM ROAST
(5 oz. meat)

1 6-lb. loin-end fresh ham
2 buds garlic

3 onions, chopped

Preheat oven to 275°. Have ham boned. Fill cavity with chopped onions and tie. Before roasting, peel garlic buds and poke into the fat on the top of the roast at 2 different places. Roast, fat side up, on rack in shallow roasting pan, uncovered. Allow 1 hour per pound. Serves 12.

BARBECUED HAM STEAKS
(6 oz. meat, 1 fat, 1 fruit)

¼ cup melted margarine
4 cups sherry wine
4 tsp. powdered cloves
½ cup dry mustard

½ cup diet brown sugar
4 tsp. paprika
8 cloves garlic, finely chopped
6 1-in. thick ham steaks

Combine ingredients and marinate ham steaks overnight. Broil 20 minutes, turning frequently and basting with marinade. Serves 6.

SCALLOPED HAM AND POTATOES
(2 bread, 2 oz. meat, 1 milk)

1 Tbs. margarine
4 cups sliced raw potatoes
Salt and pepper to taste
1 ½ cups cooked cubed ham

1 Tbs. minced onion
1 can mushroom soup
1 ¼ cups evaporated skim milk

Preheat oven to 375°. Grease a casserole with 1 tsp. margarine and place half the potatoes in casserole. Dot with 1 tsp. margarine and sprinkle with salt and pepper. Add layer of ham and onion. Top with rest of potatoes. Mix soup with milk and pour over ham and potatoes. Dot with remaining margarine and again sprinkle with salt and pepper. Cover and bake for 45 minutes. Uncover and bake 30 minutes longer, or until potatoes are browned. Serves 8.

PORK CHOP GUMBO
(3 oz. meat, 2 bread)

6 pork chops
2 ½ cups water
3 beef bouillon cubes
1 tsp. salt
½ tsp. pepper

2 onions
4 cans (16 oz.) tomatoes
1 Tbs. parsley flakes
4 cans yellow wax beans
6 potatoes, whole

Brown pork chops in skillet. Add ½ cup water and drain into a large pot. Repeat this 3 or 4 more times. Remove chops and put in large pot. Add a little water to frying pan to remove the last bit of juice and put into pot. Add bouillon cubes, salt, and pepper to juice. Add onions, tomatoes, parsley, and string beans. Cover and simmer ½ hour. Add potatoes and simmer 1 hour longer. Serves 6.

ROASTED LAMB SHANKS
(3 oz. meat, 1 fat, 1 bread)

6 lamb shanks
2 Tbs. safflower or corn oil
2 cloves garlic

3 onions, sliced
1 eggplant, unpeeled, cut in cubes
1 can tomatoes

Preheat oven to 350°. Brown lamb in oil. Add garlic and brown. Place in a casserole, pouring fat from frying pan over lamb. Add onions, eggplant, and tomatoes. Cover and simmer in oven for 1 to 2 hours. Serves 6.

HAM-ASPARAGUS BAKE
(3 oz. meat, 2 bread, 1 fat, ½ milk)

1 6-oz. can evaporated skim milk
2 cups cooked rice
3 Tbs. chopped onion
1 can cream of mushroom soup
2 cups cooked ham, cubed

1 10-oz. pkg. frozen asparagus, cooked
½ cup cornflakes
3 Tbs. melted margarine

Preheat oven to 350°. Combine milk, rice, onion, and soup. Add liquid from cooked asparagus spears to ham until very moist. Place half of ham mixture in casserole. Place asparagus spears on top. Add rest of ham mixture. Sauté corn-flakes in margarine, crush, and place on top. Bake 25 to 30 minutes. Serves 4.

LAMB PAPRIKASH
(3 oz. meat, 2 fat, 2 bread, 1 milk)

1 ½ —2 lbs. lean lamb, cut in 1-in. cubes
1 ½ Tbs. corn oil
2 cups cut-up tomatoes
1 cup chopped onion

3 Tbs. minced parsley
1 tsp. salt
½ tsp. paprika
1 cup diet sour cream
2 cups hot cooked noodles

Brown lamb cubes in hot corn oil in a heavy skillet. Add drained tomatoes, reserving ¼ cup of juice. Add onion, parsley, salt, and paprika. Cover and simmer for 1 ½ hours or until meat is tender. Skim off excess fat. Stir in imitation sour cream and reserved tomato juice. Cook over low heat until just hot. Do not boil. Serve immediately over hot noodles. Serves 6—8.

LUSCIOUS LAMB CASSEROLE
(3 oz. meat, 1 bread, 1 fat)

2 lbs. lean lamb, cut in 1-in. cubes
1—2 Tbs. corn or safflower oil
¼ cup flour
1 cup diced potatoes
½ cup diced celery
2 Tbs. catsup
1 tsp. Worcestershire sauce

2 onions, diced
1 carrot, diced
2 Tbs. minced parsley
¼ tsp. pepper
1 ½ tsp. salt
1 cup canned peas, drained

Preheat oven to 350°. Sauté lamb in oil. Drain and roll in flour. Place in casserole. Add rest of ingredients except peas. Bake in oven until meat is tender. Add peas just before serving. Serves 6—8.

PAELLA
(5 oz. meat, 1 fat, 1 bread)

3 lbs. chicken, cut up
¼ cup safflower oil
8 slices onion, 1/8-inch thick
4 medium tomatoes, cut up
1 ½ cups uncooked rice
3 cups chicken broth
2 Tbs. paprika
2 tsp. salt
½ tsp. pepper

¼ tsp. cayenne
⅛ tsp. saffron
1 cup cleaned shrimp
1 lb. fish fillets, cubed
1 5-oz. can lobster
1 package frozen peas
1 can artichoke hearts, drained
1 jar sliced pimentos, drained

Brown chicken in oil in a large pan. Remove chicken. Pour off fat from pan, add onion and tomatoes, and cook and stir for 5 minutes. Stir in rice, broth, and seasonings. Add chicken, cover pan tightly, and simmer 20 minutes. Stir in shrimp, fish, lobster, and peas. Cover and simmer 15 minutes. Gently stir in artichoke hearts and pimento. Serves 8.

BARBECUED CHICKEN WITH MUSHROOMS
(3 oz. meat, 1 fat)

1 3-lb. chicken, cut in pieces and skinned	½ tsp. pepper
	¾ tsp. chili powder
¼ cup safflower oil	1 cup catsup
2 cups water	¼ cup vinegar
1 tsp. salt	1 can mushrooms

Preheat oven to 325°. Brown chicken slowly in oil. Transfer to a roasting pan. Combine water with salt, pepper, chili powder, catsup, vinegar, mushrooms, and mushroom juice. Bring to a boil and pour over chicken in roasting pan. Bake in oven, covered, for 1 ½ hours or until chicken is done. Serves 4.

CHICKEN CASSEROLE
(4 oz. meat, 2 bread, 1 fat)

1 cup finely chopped green peppers	1 can mushroom soup
½ cup finely chopped celery	½ cup skim milk
2 small onions, chopped fine	½ cup chopped almonds
1 Tbs. safflower oil	1 pkg. frozen peas
4 cups cooked chicken	1 3-oz. can chow mein noodles

Preheat oven to 350°. Cook peppers, celery, and onions in safflower oil until tender. Add chicken, soup, milk, almonds, and peas to pepper mixture. Place half of the noodles in an ungreased casserole and pour chicken mixture over noodles. Sprinkle rest of noodles on top of chicken mixture. Bake, uncovered, in oven for 45 minutes. Serves 4.

BROILED SALMON STEAKS WITH SAUCE
(5 oz. meat, 1 fat, ¼ milk)

2 lbs. salmon steaks	1 tsp. minced parsley
Salt and pepper to taste	1 large cucumber, peeled,
⅔ cup plain yogurt	seeded, and grated
¼ cup salad dressing or diet mayonnaise	Radish roses
1 tsp. dill weed	Parsley sprigs

Sprinkle steaks with salt and pepper. Broil until tender, about 12 minutes. Blend yogurt, salad dressing, dill, minced parsley, and cucumber to make sauce. Arrange cooked salmon on a serving platter and garnish with radishes and parsley. Pass sauce separately. Serves 4.

DELICIOUS RED SNAPPER
(6 oz. meat, 1 fat)

5—6 lbs. red snapper fillets
Salt and pepper to taste
4 Tbs. lemon juice
3 Tbs. diet margarine
½ cup chopped celery

⅔ cup chopped onion
½ cup chopped green pepper
1 ½ cups (1 12-oz. can) vegetable juice
    cocktail

Preheat oven to 350°. Place fish in greased baking pan. Season with salt and pepper. Sprinkle with 2 Tbs. lemon juice and dot with 2 Tbs. margarine. Bake in oven about 25 minutes. In a saucepan, combine celery, onion, and green pepper with vegetable juice and simmer, uncovered, 15 minutes. Remove fish from oven and sprinkle with remaining lemon juice. Pour sauce over fish and dot with remaining margarine. Return to oven and bake 40 minutes more, or until fish flakes easily. Serves 10.

TURKEY GUMBO
(3 oz. meat, 2 bread)

1 turkey carcass
2 qts. water
1 Tbs. salt
1 bay leaf
2 cups chopped onion
1 cup chopped celery
1 cup chopped green pepper
1 clove garlic, minced
2 Tbs. diet margarine
1 Tbs. flour

1 16-oz. can tomatoes
¼ cup minced parsley
1 Tbs. sugar
1 tsp. Worcestershire sauce
1 10-oz. package frozen cut okra
4 cups diced turkey meat
2 cups shelled, peeled, and
    deveined shrimp
3 cups hot cooked rice

Place turkey carcass in a large soup kettle with water, salt, and bay leaf. Cover and bring to a boil. Reduce heat and simmer for 2 hours. Remove carcass and strain broth.

In a heavy skillet, cook onion, celery, green pepper, and garlic in margarine for 5 to 10 minutes, stirring constantly. Blend in flour until flour is slightly browned. Stir vegetable mixture into broth in soup kettle. Add tomatoes, parsley, sugar, and Worcestershire sauce. Bring to a boil; reduce heat and simmer 1 hour. Add okra and cook 5 minutes. Add diced turkey and shrimp. Cook slowly for 8 minutes longer.

To serve, ladle the turkey gumbo into a large soup bowl over rice. Serves 12.

LAMB RAGOUT
(3 oz. meat, 1 fat)

2 ½ lbs. lamb shoulder, cut up
½ cup diet margarine
Salt and pepper to taste
Chopped parsley
1—2 small onions, chopped fine

1 clove garlic
3 medium tomatoes, peeled and diced,
    or 1 lb. canned tomatoes
1 tsp. sugar
½ cup hot water

Cut lamb into serving pieces. Sauté in margarine until slightly browned. Add salt and pepper, parsley, onions, and garlic. Cook for a few minutes. Add tomatoes, sugar, and water. Cover and cook over low heat until lamb is tender and sauce is thick. Serve with rice. Serves 5.

MARINATED LAMB
(3 oz. meat, 1 fat, ½ fruit)

3 lbs. lean lamb, cubed
½ cup pineapple juice
¼ cup safflower oil
Juice of 1 lemon
1 tsp. salt
½ tsp. pepper

¼ tsp. sage
½ tsp. dry mustard
⅛ tsp. oregano
1 onion, chopped
1 green pepper, chopped
1 clove garlic, minced

Combine all ingredients and marinate overnight, turning lamb a few times. Drain, put lamb on skewers and broil over charcoal grill, or place on pan and broil in oven, for 20 to 30 minutes or until tender. Serves 6.

STUFFED PEPPERS
(4 oz. meat, 1 bread, 1 fat)

10 to 12 medium-size green peppers
2 tsp. salt
¼ cup diet margarine
1 onion, finely chopped
1 clove garlic
1 ½ lbs. ground beef

½ cup cooked rice
2−3 Tbs. chopped parsley
2 tomatoes, peeled and chopped
Salt and pepper to taste
¾ cup soft bread crumbs
1 ½ cups tomato juice

Preheat oven to 350°. Cut off a slice at the stem end of peppers; seed and wash. Place in boiling salted water and boil for 5 minutes. Drain. Heat half of margarine in frying pan and sauté onion until soft. Add garlic and beef, stirring with a fork. Add rice, parsley, tomatoes, and salt and pepper. Simmer for 5 minutes. Fill peppers with beef-rice mixture and replace cut-off slices as lids. Place filled peppers upright in a baking dish. Mix bread crumbs with remaining margarine and sprinkle over the top of each pepper. Pour tomato juice in baking dish around peppers. Bake in oven, uncovered, about 1 hour. Serves 6.

BEST EVER MEAT LOAF
(3 oz. meat, 1 bread)

1 ½ lbs. ground beef
¾ cup oatmeal
1 ½ tsp. salt
1 tsp. onion salt

1 tsp. celery salt
1 can tomato paste
3 Tbs. egg substitute

Preheat oven to 350°. Combine all ingredients and mix thoroughly. Pack firmly into an ungreased 8 ½ X 4 ½ X 2 ½-inch loaf pan. Bake in oven for 1 hour and 15 minutes. Let stand 5 minutes before slicing. Serves 6.

HAIWAIIAN KEBOB
(3 oz. meat, 1 bread)

2 lbs. lamb shoulder, cut in 4 pieces
2 green peppers, halved
2 tomatoes, halved
1 onion, quartered

1 medium eggplant, quartered
1 potato, quartered
Salt and pepper to taste

Preheat oven to 350°. Tear or cut 4 large squares of heavy-duty aluminum foil. In the center of each square, place 1 piece of lamb, ½ pepper, ½ tomato, ¼ onion, ¼ eggplant, and ¼ potato, and sprinkle with salt and pepper. Fold each unit into a compact package and place packages side by side in a roasting pan. Bake in oven for 3 hours. Do not turn packages; do not use water. Leave in individual packages and serve. Serves 4.

DUTCH MEAT LOAF
(3 oz. meat, 1 bread)

1 ½ lbs. ground beef
1 can condensed tomato soup
1 cup uncooked rolled oats
1 ½ tsp. salt
¼ tsp. pepper
1 medium onion, finely chopped

3 Tbs. egg substitute
2 Tbs. prepared mustard
¼ cup vinegar
¼ cup brown sugar
1 cup water

Preheat oven to 350°. In a mixing bowl, combine meat, ½ can soup, rolled oats, salt, pepper, and onion. Mix well and add egg substitute. Spoon mixture into a greased bread tin. Bake in oven for about 1 ½ hours. While it is baking, prepare sauce: Combine mustard, remaining tomato soup, vinegar, sugar, and water. Baste meat with sauce as it cooks. Serves 6.

CHEESE SPECIAL
(2 oz. meat, 1 bread)

1 slice bread
1 oz. low-cholesterol cheese

1 oz. sliced ham
1 slice tomato

Preheat oven to 350°. Place bread on baking sheet and place cheese on bread. Lay ham and then tomato slice over this. Heat in oven until cheese begins to melt and ham browns. Serves 1.

CHEESE FONDUE
(2 oz. meat, 1 bread, 1 milk)

⅓ cup egg substitute
1 cup skim milk
1 slice bread, cubed

1 oz. low-cholesterol cheese, diced
Salt and pepper to taste

Preheat oven to 375°. Beat egg substitute and add milk and cubed bread. Add diced cheese and seasoning. Place mixture in a small baking dish and bake for 20 to 30 minutes or until firm. Serves 1.

EGG AND CHEESE SUPREME
(2 oz. meat, 1 fat)

1 oz. low-cholesterol cheese	Salt and pepper to taste
1 tsp. margarine	⅓ cup egg substitute
1 small tomato, sliced	

Preheat oven to 350°. Place cheese in an oven-proof baking dish greased with margarine. Cover with tomato slices and season with salt and pepper. Beat egg substitute and pour over cheese and tomato. Bake in oven for 40 to 45 minutes. Serves 1.

SPANISH OMELET
(1 oz. meat, 1 fat)

⅓ cup egg substitute	Pinch of salt
1 ½ tsp. water	Pinch of pepper
½ tsp. chopped onion	1 tsp. margarine
½ tsp. chopped green pepper	

Beat egg until foamy. Add water, onion, green pepper, salt, and pepper. Melt margarine in frying pan and add egg mixture. After allowing to cook for a second, begin stirring and continue to cook and stir until brown. Serve at once. Serves 1.

TART CABBAGE
(1 fat)

Salt	1 tsp. horseradish
Paprika	Artificial sweetener (optional)
1 tsp. lemon juice	½ cup cooked cabbage
1 tsp. margarine	

Blend salt, paprika, lemon juice, margarine, and horseradish. Add sweetener if desired. Pour over cooked cabbage. Serves 1.

BAKED STUFFED POTATO
(1 bread, 1 fat, 1 oz. meat)

1 small potato	1 oz. low-cholesterol cheese
1 tsp. margarine	Paprika

Preheat oven to 425° and bake potato. Remove from oven and turn oven off. Cut slice from top and scoop out inside, being careful not to break shell. Mash potato pulp and add margarine and cheese while still hot. Mix well and spoon back into shell, mounding slightly. Sprinkle with paprika and replace in oven until golden brown. Serves 1.

HOBO VEGETABLES
(1 bread, 1 fat)

½ cup carrots
¼ cup sliced onions
1 small potato

½ tsp. margarine
Salt and pepper to taste

Preheat oven to 350°. Place vegetables on a piece of aluminum foil. Add margarine and seasoning. Wrap snugly and seal. Bake on oven rack for 30 to 40 minutes, until vegetables are done. Serves 1.

STUFFED ZUCCHINI
(½ oz. meat, ½ fat)

2 medium zucchini
1 tsp. crushed garlic
1 Tbs. oil
¼ cup chopped mushrooms
1 Tbs. diced onion

½ tsp. minced parsley
Dash of marjoram
Salt and pepper to taste
¼ cup egg substitute

Preheat oven to 350° and lightly oil a baking pan. Lightly scrub zucchini to remove wax or grit. Parboil for 10 minutes. Drain, cool, and cut in half lengthwise. Carefully remove zucchini pulp from shell and chop finely. Sauté garlic in oil and discard garlic. Sauté mushrooms and onion in the same oil. Add zucchini pulp, parsley, marjoram, salt and pepper. Cool. Stir in the egg substitute and fill each zucchini half with the mixture. Place stuffed halves on baking pan and bake in oven for 30 minutes. Serves 2.

TOMATO AND EGG
(1 oz. meat, 1 fat)

1 tsp. margarine
1 medium tomato
⅓ cup egg substitute

1 tsp. chopped pimento
Salt and pepper to taste

Melt margarine in a frying pan. Cut tomato in half and brown lightly. Remove from pan. Beat egg substitute and pimento together and brown in same pan until creamy. Season and serve together. Serves 1.

ONION AND APPLE CASSEROLE
(1 bread, 1 fruit, 1 fat)

4 large apples, peeled and sliced
3 large onions, sliced
1 cup bread crumbs

Salt and pepper to taste
1 Tbs. margarine
2 cups beef or chicken bouillon

Preheat oven to 350°. Place apples, onions, bread crumbs, and seasoning in a greased casserole in layers. Dot with margarine and pour on bouillon. Bake for 1 hour. Serves 4.

SCRAMBLED CABBAGE
(1 fat)

4 cups shredded cabbage
1 ½ cups canned tomatoes
1 large onion, chopped fine
½ tsp. salt
½ tsp. sugar

Dash of pepper
Bread crumbs
Grated cheese
2 Tbs. margarine

Preheat oven to 350°. Cook cabbage, tomatoes, and onion in a small amount of boiling water for about 10 minutes. Add seasonings. Garnish with bread crumbs and grated cheese. Dot with margarine. Bake in oven for 20 minutes. Serves 4.

VEGETABLE RING
(2 bread, 1 fat, ½ milk)

2 cups soft bread crumbs
2 cups skim milk
6 Tbs. egg substitute
1 tsp. salt
¼ tsp. pepper
1 8-oz. pkg. frozen peas

4 stalks celery, sliced thin
1 cup grated carrots
¼ lb. fresh mushrooms, cut up
2 Tbs. margarine
⅛ cup flour

Soak bread crumbs in 1 cup milk for ½ hour. Preheat oven to 350°. Add egg substitute, salt and pepper, and vegetables to softened bread crumbs. Pour into greased ring pan and bake in oven for 1 hour. To make sauce, sauté mushrooms in margarine. Remove mushrooms and add ⅛ cup flour to the margarine and enough skim milk to make a medium sauce. Add mushrooms and salt and pepper to taste. Serves 4.

CARROT RING
(1 fruit, 1 fat, 1 bread)

2 cups grated carrots
1 cup flour
½ cup brown sugar
½ cup melted margarine

1 tsp. baking powder
6 Tbs. egg substitute
1 tsp. salt
½ tsp. baking soda

Preheat oven to 375°. Mix all ingredients together and pour in greased ring pan. Bake in oven until set and brown, about 1 hour. Serves 4.

DESSERTS, BREADS, AND APPETIZERS

MINTED FRUIT
(1 fruit)

4 mint leaves
1 unsweetened pear half or
  ½ fresh pear

1 lettuce leaf
½ cup fresh or unsweetened frozen
  strawberries

Wash and chop mint leaves. Roll pear half in moist leaves. Place lettuce leaf on a dish and set the pear on it. Fill center with strawberries and place extra ones around pear. Chill. Serves 1.

CHEESY FRUIT
(1 oz. meat, 1 fruit)

½ cup unsweetened fruit cocktail   1 lettuce leaf
¼ cup cottage cheese

Drain fruit and blend with cottage cheese. Place in a custard cup and freeze for 45 minutes. Remove from cup and serve on lettuce leaf. Serves 1.

BROILED GRAPEFRUIT
(1 fruit, 1 fat, 1 bread)

1 grapefruit, halved   Chopped walnuts
2 oz. brandy   2 tsp. margarine

Pour brandy on grapefruit halves. Put chopped walnuts on top, a pat of margarine in center, and broil for five minutes. Serves 2.

CANTALOUPE CUP
(2 fruit)

2 cantaloupes   1 Tbs. lemon juice
1 can crushed pineapple   1 cup green grapes

Scoop pulp of cantaloupes and cut into cubes. Add crushed pineapple and lemon juice. Add green grapes if in season. Chill. Serves 8.

APPLE CLOUD
(1 fruit)

1 pkg. diet lemon gelatin   ½ cup unsweetened applesauce
½ cup hot water

Dissolve gelatin in hot water. Chill until syrupy. Set the bowl in another larger bowl of ice. Beat until fluffy. Fold in applesauce. Place in a dessert glass. Chill. Serves 1

FRUITY TAPIOCA
(1 fruit, ½ bread)

1 Tbs. quick-cooking tapioca   ½ cup unsweetened fruit juice

Mix together tapioca and fruit juice. Boil over a low flame for 1 to 2 minutes. Cool and serve. Serves 1.

CREAMED GELATIN
(¼ milk)

1 pkg. unsweetened gelatin
1 cup boiling water
½ cup cold water

1 cup skim milk
3 tsp. liquid sweetener
(2 Tbs. sugar substitute)

Dissolve gelatin in boiling water. Add cold water and chill until nearly firm. Beat milk with gelatin mixture. Add sugar substitute and chill. Break chilled mixture up. Beat until fluffy. Chill until set. Serve within 4 hours. Serves 4.

JEAN'S BAKED APPLES
(1 fruit, ½ fat)

1 apple
1 Tbs. diet margarine
2 Tbs. sugar substitute

½ tsp. cinnamon
1 Tbs. low-calorie topping

Preheat oven to 300°. Core apple. Put margarine, sugar substitute, and cinnamon in cavity. Place in baking dish and add water to cover bottom of dish. Bake in oven for 30 minutes or until tender. Serve with topping. Serves 1.

APPLE CASSEROLE
(2 fruit, 1 bread, ½ fat)

½ cup diet margarine
3 cups Corn Chex
4 apples
½ cup raisins

½ tsp. cinnamon
½ cup sugar substitute
1 Tbs. lemon juice
1 Tbs. low-calorie topping

Preheat oven to 350°. Melt margarine and pour over cereal. Put aside. Cut up and core apples, add raisins, and put aside. In another bowl, mix cinnamon, sugar substitute, and lemon juice. Layer bottom of casserole with ⅓ of cereal. Add ½ of the apples and raisins. Sprinkle ½ of sugar mixture over apples, and repeat. Top layer should be cereal. Bake in oven covered for 20 minutes and uncovered for 20 minutes more. Serve hot with topping. Serves 4–6.

APPLE CHEESE CAKE
(1 oz. meat, 1 fruit, 2 fat, 2 bread)

½ cup margarine
½ cup sugar
1 cup flour
¼ tsp. vanilla
1 4-oz. pkg. imitation
    cream cheese

1 cup cottage cheese
3 Tbs. egg substitute
2 large apples, diced
¼ cup sliced almonds
½ cup cinnamon

Preheat oven to 400°. Make crust by mixing margarine, ¼ cup sugar, flour, and vanilla in large bowl. Pat dough in bottom of 9-inch pie pan. Blend cheeses and egg substitute in blender and pour into crust. Mix apples, almonds, ¼ cup sugar, and cinnamon and sprinkle over top. Bake in oven for 35 minutes. Serves 10.

BLUEBERRY PIE
(1 fruit, ½ meat)

Thin pie crust to fit 5-in. plate	1 tsp. plain gelatin
1 cup blueberries	1 Tbs. water

Roll out pie crust and bake according to pie crust directions. Heat berries over a moderate flame. Place gelatin in a bowl and add water to soften. Add berries. Mix well and pour into crust. Cool. Refrigerate. Yields 2 servings.

QUICK LEMON CAKE
(1 bread, 1 oz. meat, 1 fat)

⅓ cup egg substitute	⅛ tsp. lemon rind
2 Tbs. lemon juice	1 angel food cake cut
½ cup water	into 1-inch sections
1 pkg. unsweetened lemon gelatin	3 Tbs. low-cholesterol creamer

Mix egg substitute with lemon juice and water. Cook in double boiler until mixture is thick enough to coat a spoon. Dissolve gelatin in mixture and add lemon rind. Cut cake into bite-size pieces and fold into mixture. Spoon into parfait glasses and chill for 24 hours. Top with whipped creamer. Serves 12.

STRAWBERRY SHORTCAKE
(1 bread, 1 fruit, 1 fat)

1 cup unsweetened or fresh strawberries	3 Tbs. low-cholesterol creamer
	1 2-in. baking powder biscuit

Split the biscuit. Slice berries and place on biscuit. Beat creamer and cover berries. Serves 1.

ORANGE COOKIES
(5 cookies = 1 bread, 2 fat)

1 ¾ tsp. liquid sweetener	1 cup flour
¼ cup unsweetened orange juice	¼ tsp. salt
1 tsp. vanilla	¼ tsp. baking powder
4 Tbs. margarine	

Blend sweetener, orange juice, and vanilla. Cream margarine. Sift dry ingredients together. Add to liquid mixture and margarine. Shape dough into roll approximately 15 inches long; wrap in wax paper. Chill until firm. Preheat oven to 400°. Cut dough into ⅛-inch-thick slices. Place on cookie sheet and bake about 10 minutes or until golden brown. Makes 30 cookies.

ICEBOX COOKIES
(5 cookies = 1 bread, 3 fat)

1 cup margarine
½ tsp. liquid sweetener
⅓ cup egg substitute

2 ½ cups flour
1 tsp. vanilla
Cinnamon (optional)

Cream margarine. Add sweetener, then add egg substitute and mix well. Sift flour and add, mixing well. Add vanilla and blend. Form into a roll about 16 inches long. Wrap in wax paper and chill in refrigerator overnight.

Preheat oven to 350°. Slice roll ¼ inch thick and place slices on cookie sheet. Sprinkle with cinnamon, if desired. Bake 8–10 minutes or until brown. Makes 60 cookies.

STRIPED CEREAL COOKIES
(5 cookies = 2 bread, 1 fat, 1 oz. meat)

1 cup sugar
¾ cup margarine
2 eggs or ½ cup egg substitute
1 tsp. vanilla
2 ½ cups all-purpose flour

½ tsp. baking soda
2 cups Rice Crispies, crushed
2 squares semisweet chocolate,
    melted and cooled

Beat together sugar and margarine. Add eggs and vanilla and mix until light and fluffy. Stir flour and soda into egg mixture. Stir in Rice Crispies. Divide dough in half. Add cooled chocolate to half of dough. Line bottom of an 8 X 4 X 2 loaf pan with waxed paper. Press ½ chocolate dough into pan; top with ½ plain dough. Repeat. Cover and refrigerate until firm, about 5 hours. Preheat oven to 375°. Remove dough from pan. Cut loaf crosswise into thirds. Cut crosswise in thin slices. Place on ungreased cookie sheet. Bake in oven for 10 to 12 minutes until done. Makes 60 cookies.

SOUR CREAM BRAN COOKIES
(2 cookies = 2 fruit, 1 oz. meat, 2 bread, 1 fat)

½ cup margarine
½ cup sugar
½ cup brown sugar
1 egg or ¼ cup egg substitute
½ cup imitation sour cream
1 tsp. vanilla

1 ¾ cups all-purpose flour
½ tsp. baking soda
½ tsp. salt
1 cup bran flakes
½ cup raisins or coconut

Preheat oven to 375°. Cream margarine, sugar, and brown sugar until fluffy. Add egg, sour cream, and vanilla and beat. Stir flour, soda, and salt into creamed mixture. Fold in bran flakes and raisins or coconut. Drop by rounded teaspoonfuls onto greased cookie sheet. Bake in oven for 10 to 12 minutes. Makes 30 cookies.

WHEAT TWIST
(3 bread)

¾ cup apple juice
⅓ cup wheat germ
2 pkgs. dry yeast
¼ cup warm water
3 Tbs. margarine, softened

¼ cup honey
2 tsp. salt
3 Tbs. egg substitute
2¾ —3 cups white flour
1 cup whole wheat flour

Heat apple juice to boiling in small saucepan. Stir in wheat germ and cool. Dissolve yeast in warm water in large mixing bowl. Stir in margarine, honey, salt, egg substitute, wheat germ and apple juice mixture, and 2 cups of white flour. Beat until smooth.

Divide dough in half. Stir in enough of the whole wheat flour to ½ of dough to form a soft dough. Stir in enough of the remaining white flour to other ½ to form a soft dough. Turn each half onto lightly floured surface and knead until smooth and elastic, about 5 minutes. Place in greased bowls, turn greased sides up. Cover; let rise in warm place until double, about 1 ½ hours. (Dough is ready if an indentation remains when touched.)

Punch down dough; roll each half into a rope about 16 inches long. Place ropes side by side on greased baking sheet; twist together gently and loosely. Pinch ends to fasten. Let rise until double (1 hour). Heat oven to 350°. Bake until twist is done, 30 to 35 minutes. Serves 8.

HEALTH BREAD
(1 fat, 3 bread, 1 meat)

6 ¼ to 6 ½ cups white flour
1 cup whole wheat flour
2 pkgs. dry yeast
1 cup quick-cooking rolled oats
1 cup whole bran cereal

2 ½ cups boiling water
1 ½ cups diet cottage cheese
2 Tbs. margarine
½ cup honey
2 Tbs. salt

In large mixing bowl, thoroughly stir together 2 cups white flour, whole wheat flour, and yeast. In another bowl, combine oats, bran, boiling water, cottage cheese, margarine, honey, and salt; stir mixture constantly until margarine melts. Add honey mixture to dry ingredients in bowl. Beat ½ minute at low speed with electric mixer, scraping sides of bowl constantly. Beat 3 minutes at high speed. By hand, stir in enough of remaining flour to make a moderately stiff dough. Turn out onto lightly floured surface. Knead until smooth and elastic, 5 to 7 minutes. Place in greased bowl, turning over to grease entire surface. Cover and let rise in warm place till double (1 hour).

Punch dough down; divide into thirds. Cover and let rest 10 minutes. Shape each portion into a loaf. Place in 3 greased 8½ × 4½ × 2½-inch loaf pans. Cover and let rise until double, 35 to 45 minutes. Heat oven to 375°. Bake loaves for 35 to 45 minutes. Serves 8.

APPLE BRAN CASSEROLE BREAD
(3 bread, 1 fruit, ½ fat)

3 cups flour
1 cup whole bran
1 pkg. dry yeast
1 cup water

1 8-oz. can (1 cup) applesauce
¼ cup margarine
2 Tbs. brown sugar
1 tsp. salt

In a large mixing bowl combine 1½ cups flour, bran, and yeast. In a saucepan, heat water, applesauce, margarine, sugar, and salt until just warm, stirring to melt margarine. Add to dry mixture in bowl. Beat at low speed of electric mixer ½ minute, scraping sides of bowl constantly. Beat 3 minutes at high speed. By hand, stir in remaining flour to make a soft dough. Beat well. Cover and let rise in warm place until double in size (about 1 hour).

Punch dough down. Turn into greased 2-quart casserole. Let rise in warm place until double (about 40 minutes). Heat oven to 350°. Brush bread with a little melted margarine and bake in oven for 55 minutes. Cover with foil the last 15 minutes of baking time. Remove from casserole; cool on rack. Serves 8.

BANANA BREAD
(1 fruit, 1 bread, 1 fat)

1½ cup mashed ripe bananas
¼ cup safflower oil
½ cup honey
6 Tbs. egg substitute,
  slightly beaten

1 tsp. vanilla
2 cups whole wheat flour
¼ cup wheat germ
1 tsp. salt
1 tsp. baking soda

Preheat oven to 350°. Mix bananas, oil, honey, egg substitute, and vanilla. Mix flour, wheat germ, salt, and soda. Add dry ingredients to banana mixture in 2 or 3 parts, beating well until smooth. Place batter in an oiled 9 × 5 × 3-inch loaf pan (or 2 smaller pans) and bake for about 1 hour. Cool before slicing. Serves 8.

FRUIT KABOBS
(1 fruit)

1⅛-in. wedge cantaloupe
½ cup watermelon

Unsweetened lemon juice
Fresh mint

Scoop out melon into ball shapes. Marinate in lemon juice for 1 hour. Alternate balls on skewers. Serve garnished with fresh mint. Serves 1.

CRUNCHY CEREAL
(1 bread, 2 fat)

½ cup wheat squares, rice squares,   ¼ tsp celery salt
   corn squares, or puffed cereal   ¼ tsp. onion salt
1 Tbs. oil   8 peanuts
¾ tsp. Worcestershire sauce

Heat oven to 275°. Combine cereals. In a saucepan, warm oil and add Worcestershire sauce and seasonings. Add to cereal mixture. Add peanuts and mix. Place in a shallow pan; bake for 1 hour. Stir every 10 minutes. Serves 1.

VEGETABLE BED
(free)

Asparagus spears   Cherry tomatoes
Broccoli florets   Cucumber slices
Carrot strips   Green pepper strips
Cauliflower florets   Radish roses
Celery sticks   Turnip wedges

Arrange a few of each vegetable on a platter. Serve with chili sauce or cucumber dip.

CHILI SAUCE DIP
(free)

1 12-oz. bottle chili sauce   2 Tbs. horseradish
2 Tbs. lemon juice   ¼ cup chopped green pepper
3 drops tabasco sauce   1 ½ Tbs. minced parsley

Combine ingredients and chill. Serve with vegetable bed.

CUCUMBER DIP
(1 fat, ⅓ milk)

1 medium cucumber, peeled and   1 tsp. vinegar
   finely chopped   ½ tsp. salt
1 cup yogurt   1 tsp. chopped dill
1 tsp. olive oil   1 clove garlic, minced
1 tsp. safflower oil

Combine all ingredients and chill for at least 1 hour. Serve as a dip with fresh vegetables. Serves 6.

CUCUMBER AND YOGURT DIP
(½ milk, 1 bread)

1 small cucumber   Onion powder to taste
½ cup plain yogurt   Dash of Worcestershire sauce

Wash cucumber, grate, and drain well until almost dry. Combine with yogurt, onion powder, and Worcestershire sauce. Serve with crackers. Serves 1.

POVERTY CAVIAR
(1 fat, 1 bread)

1 small eggplant
1 Tbs. vegetable oil
2 tsp. chopped onion
½ tsp. minced garlic

⅛ cup chopped green pepper
2 tsp. lemon juice
Salt and pepper to taste
Chopped parsley

Slice eggplant in half and rub with 1 ½ tsp. oil. Place halves cut side down on baking pan. Broil on middle rack in oven or lower rack in broiler for 20 to 25 minutes, or until soft. Cool slightly. Scoop out pulp and mash with fork. Sauté onion and garlic in remaining oil. Stir into eggplant pulp. Add green pepper, lemon juice, and salt and pepper. Chill 2 hours. Sprinkle with parsley. Serve with Melba Rounds. Serves 4.

CUCUMBER BOWL
(free)

1 cucumber
Chopped celery
Chopped tomato

Chopped green pepper
Vinegar
Lettuce leaf

Wash cucumber and cut an oblong piece off one side. Continue to scoop out cucumber until it resembles a canoe. Fill with a mixture of celery, tomato, and green pepper with vinegar. Set on lettuce leaf. Serves 1.

CUCUMBER CANAPÉ
(1 bread)

1 small cucumber, sliced thin
Low-calorie oil and vinegar dressing

Toasted bread rounds
Green pepper or pimento slice

Marinate cucumber slices in dressing. Place slices of cucumber on toasted bread rounds and decorate with green pepper or pimento. Serves 1.

MUSHROOM CANAPÉ
(free)

1 can button mushrooms
Diet French dressing

Chopped parsley

Marinate mushrooms in French dressing. Roll in parsley and serve on toothpicks. Serves 4.

TUNA SPREAD
(1 meat, 1 fat)

1 7 oz. can tuna, packed in water
½ cup celery, diced
¼ cup diet mayonnaise

1 Tbs. lemon juice
Onion powder
Salt and pepper to taste

Mix all ingredients together and season with onion powder, salt, and pepper. Serves 4.

MOCK CHOPPED LIVER
(1 meat, 1 fat, 1 bread)

3 hard-boiled eggs or 9 Tbs.
  egg substitute, scrambled
2 large onions, sliced and sautéed

1 small can mushrooms
12 walnuts, shelled
Salt and pepper to taste

Grind ingredients together and season with salt and pepper. Spread on rye bread or crackers. Serves 3.

YOGURT DIP
(1 Tbs. = 1 fat)

1 Tbs. safflower oil
1 clove garlic, put through
  a garlic press

¼ cup diced cucumber
⅛ cup diced radishes
1 cup yogurt

Mix all ingredients and use as a dip with raw vegetables or crackers.

HOT CRABMEAT DIP
(2 meat, 3 fat)

1 can crabmeat
1 8-oz. pkg. imitation cream cheese
¼ cup lemon juice
1 small onion, grated

½ tsp. prepared horseradish
Dash of Worcestershire sauce
Garlic salt to taste
Slivered almonds

Preheat oven to 400°. Mix crabmeat and cheese with lemon juice, onion, and seasonings and place in casserole. Sprinkle with slivered almonds. Bake in oven until bubbling and lightly browned. Serve with crackers. Serves 12.

IMITATION SOUR CREAM
(1 Tbs. = 1 fat)

1 Tbs. lemon juice
¼ cup water

¼ tsp. salt
⅔ cup cottage cheese

Mix ingredients and chill. Makes 1 cup.
  For dips, add cut-up cucumbers, green onions, radishes, green pepper, and

salt and pepper to taste. Or add cut-up anchovies, capers, and chopped parsley.

For salad dressings, add 1 garlic bud, pressed in garlic press or chopped fine, and a dash of cayenne and paprika. Or add chopped chives or dill weed.

Appendix

COMPOSITION OF FOODS
100 GRAMS OR 3.5 OUNCES
(EDIBLE PORTION)

Food and Description	Water %	Calories	Protein	Fat	Carbo-hydrate Total†	Fiber Only
Anchovy						
pickled	58.6	176	19.2	10.3	.3	0
Apples						
raw	84.4	58	.2	.6	14.5	1.0
Apple juice						
canned or bottled	87.8	47	.1	trace	11.9	.1
Applesauce, canned						
unsweetened	88.5	41	.2	.2	10.8	.6
sweetened	75.7	91	.2	.1	23.8	.5
Apricots						
raw	85.3	51	1.0	.2	12.8	.6
Artichokes						
cooked, boiled	86.5	40	2.8	.2	9.9	2.4
Asparagus						
cooked spears, boiled	93.6	20	2.2	.2	3.6	.7
Bananas						
common	75.7	85	1.1	.2	22.2	.5
Barley, pearled						
light	11.1	349	8.2	1.0	78.8	.5
pot or scotch	10.8	348	9.6	1.1	77.2	.4
Bass, striped						
cooked, oven-fried	60.8	196	21.5	8.5	6.7	—
Beans, lima						
cooked, boiled	71.1	111	7.6	.5	19.8	1.8
Beans, snap						
canned						
solids and liquid	93.5	18	1.0	.1	4.2	.6
yellow or wax						
cooked, boiled	93.4	22	1.4	.2	4.6	1.0
Beef						
carcass						
prime grade						
(54% lean, 46% fat)	44.8	428	13.6	41.0	0	0
choice grade						
(60% lean, 40% fat)	49.4	379	14.9	35.0	0	0

†Sugars, starches, and fiber

Food and Description	Water %	Calories	Protein	Fat	Carbo-hydrate Total†	Fiber Only
Beef cont'd						
utility grade						
(76% lean, 24% fat)	62.5	242	18.6	18.0	0	0
retail cuts						
chuck cuts						
cooked, braised						
(81% lean, 19% fat)	49.4	327	26.0	23.9	0	0
london broil						
cooked, braised						
(100% lean)	61.4	196	30.5	7.3	0	0
loin or short loin						
porterhouse steak						
cooked, broiled						
(57% lean, 43% fat)	37.2	465	19.7	42.2	0	0
t-bone steak						
cooked, broiled						
(56% lean, 44% fat)	36.4	473	19.5	43.2	0	0
club steak						
cooked, broiled						
(58% lean, 42% fat)	37.9	454	20.6	40.6	0	0
loin end or sirloin						
sirloin steak						
cooked, broiled						
(66% lean, 34% fat)	43.9	387	23.0	32.0	0	0
double-bone sirloin						
steak cooked,						
broiled						
(66% lean, 34% fat)	42.1	408	22.2	34.7	0	0
round, entire						
cooked, broiled						
(81% lean, 19% fat)	54.7	261	28.6	15.4	0	0
hamburger, ground						
beef lean, cooked	60.0	219	27.4	11.3	0	0
regular ground						
cooked	54.2	286	24.2	20.3	0	0
Beef						
canned, roast beef	60.0	224	25.0	13.0	0	0
Beef, corned						
cooked, medium-fat	43.9	372	22.9	30.4	0	0

†Sugars, starches, and fiber

Food and Description	Water %	Calories	Protein	Fat	Carbo-hydrate Total†	Fiber Only
Beets, common red						
cooked, boiled	90.9	32	1.1	.1	7.2	.8
Beverages, alcoholic						
beer	92.1	42	.3	0	3.8	—
86 proof	64.0	249	—	—	trace	—
90 proof	62.1	263	—	—	trace	—
wine						
table	85.6	85	.1	0	4.2	—
carbonated						
sweetened	92.0	31	*	*	8.0	*
cola type	90.0	39	*	*	10.0	*
ginger ale	92.0	31	*	*	8.0	*
Blackberries	84.5	58	1.2	.9	12.9	4.1
Blueberries						
raw	83.2	62	.7	.5	15.3	1.5
Bonito	67.6	168	24.0	7.3	0	0
Bran flakes	3.0	303	10.2	1.8	80.6	3.6
Breads						
cracked wheat	34.9	263	8.7	2.2	52.1	.5
French or vienna	30.6	290	9.1	3.0	55.4	.2
Italian	31.8	276	9.1	3.8	56.4	.2
pumpernickel	34.0	246	9.1	1.2	53.1	1.1
white	35.8	269	8.7	3.2	50.4	.2
whole wheat	36.4	243	10.5	3.0	47.7	1.6
Bread crumbs	6.5	392	12.6	4.6	73.4	.3
Broccoli						
cooked, boiled	91.3	26	3.1	.3	4.5	1.5
Brussels sprouts						
cooked, boiled	88.2	36	4.2	.4	6.4	1.6
Butter	15.5	716	.6	81.0	.4	0
Buttermilk						
fluid	90.5	36	3.6	.1	5.1	0
Cabbage						
cooked, boiled	93.9	20	1.1	.2	4.3	.8
Cakes						
chocolate						
without icing	24.6	366	4.8	17.2	52.0	.3

†Sugars, starches, and fiber
*Too low to measure.

Food and Description	Water %	Calories	Protein	Fat	Carbo-hydrate Total†	Fiber Only
Cakes cont'd						
with chocolate icing	22.0	369	4.5	16.4	55.8	.3
with white icing	21.3	369	3.8	14.6	59.2	.2
fruitcake						
dark	18.1	379	4.8	15.3	59.7	.6
plain cake or cupcake						
without icing	24.5	364	4.5	13.9	55.9	.1
with chocolate icing	21.4	368	4.2	13.9	59.4	.2
pound						
old-fashioned	17.2	473	5.7	29.5	47.0	.1
Candy						
butterscotch	1.5	397	trace	3.4	94.8	0
chocolate-coated						
almonds	2.0	569	12.3	43.7	39.6	1.5
fudge						
chocolate	8.2	400	2.7	12.2	75.0	.2
marshmallows	17.3	319	2.0	trace	80.4	0
peanut bars	1.5	515	17.5	32.2	47.2	1.2
Carrots						
canned, regular						
pack, solids, liquids	91.8	28	.6	.2	6.5	.6
Cashew nuts	5.2	561	17.2	45.7	29.3	1.4
Cauliflower						
cooked, boiled	92.8	22	2.3	.2	4.1	1.0
Celery						
raw	94.1	17	.9	.1	3.9	.6
cooked, boiled	95.3	14	.8	.1	3.1	.6
Cheeses						
brick	41.0	370	22.2	30.5	1.9	0
cottage						
uncreamed	79.0	86	17.0	.3	2.7	0
Parmesan	30.0	393	36.0	26.0	2.9	0
Swiss, domestic	39.0	370	27.5	28.0	1.7	0
Cherries						
raw						
sour, red	83.7	58	1.2	.3	14.3	.2
Chicken						
light meat						
cooked, roasted	63.8	166	31.6	3.4	0	0
broilers, broiled	71.0	136	23.8	3.8	0	0

†Sugars, starches, and fiber

Food and Description	Water %	Calories	Protein	Fat	Carbo-hydrate Total†	Fiber Only
roasters						
cooked, roasted	62.8	183	29.5	6.3	0	0
canned	65.2	198	21.7	11.7	0	0
Chocolate						
bitter or baking	2.3	505	10.7	53.0	28.9	2.5
Chop suey, with meat						
cooked, home recipe	75.4	120	10.4	6.8	5.1	.5
Chow mein, chicken						
cooked, home recipe	78.0	102	12.4	4.0	4.0	.3
Clams, raw						
meat and liquid	86.2	49	6.5	.4	4.2	—
Cod						
cooked, broiled	64.6	170	28.5	5.3	0	0
Coleslaw						
mayonnaise	79.0	144	1.3	14.0	4.8	.7
Cookies						
chocolate	4.0	445	7.1	15.7	71.5	.3
chocolate chip, home						
recipe	3.0	516	5.4	30.1	60.1	.4
oatmeal with raisins	2.8	451	6.2	15.4	73.5	.4
Corn, sweet						
raw, white and yellow	72.7	96	3.5	1.0	22.1	.7
cooked, boiled	76.5	83	3.2	1.0	18.8	.7
Corn grits, degermed						
dry	12.0	362	8.7	.8	78.1	.4
Cornflakes	3.8	386	7.9	.4	85.3	.7
Cornbread, home recipe	53.9	207	7.4	7.2	29.1	.5
spoon bread	63.0	195	6.7	11.4	16.9	.3
Crab, canned	77.2	101	17.4	2.5	1.1	—
Crackers						
cheese	3.9	479	11.2	21.3	60.4	.2
Cream, fluid						
heavy whipping	56.6	352	2.2	37.6	3.1	0
Cucumbers, raw	95.1	15	.9	.1	3.4	.6
Dates, dry	22.5	274	2.2	.5	72.9	2.3
Doughnuts						
cake type	23.7	391	4.6	18.6	51.4	.1
yeast leavened	28.3	414	6.3	26.7	37.7	.2

†Sugars, starches, and fiber

Food and Description	Water %	Calories	Protein	Fat	Carbo-hydrate Total†	Fiber Only
Duck	68.8	165	21.4	8.2	0	0
Eggs, chicken						
whole, fresh, frozen	73.7	163	12.9	11.5	.9	0
yolks, fresh	51.1	348	16.0	30.6	.6	0
cooked, fried	67.7	216	13.8	17.2	.3	0
Eggplant						
cooked, boiled	94.3	19	1.0	.2	4.1	.9
Farina						
cooked	89.5	42	1.3	.1	8.7	trace
Fats						
cooking, vegetable fat	0	884	0	100.0	0	0
Fish sticks,						
frozen, cooked	65.8	176	16.6	8.9	6.5	—
Flat fishes						
sole, flounder, raw	81.3	79	16.7	.8	0	0
Flounder						
cooked, baked	58.1	202	30.0	8.2	0	0
Fruit cocktail						
water pack	89.6	37	.4	.1	9.7	.4
syrup pack						
extra heavy	75.6	92	.4	.1	23.7	.4
Garlic						
cloves, raw	61.3	137	6.2	.2	30.8	1.5
Grapefruit raw						
all varieties	88.4	41	.5	.1	10.6	.2
juice, all varieties	90.0	39	.5	.1	9.2	trace
Haddock						
cooked, fried	66.3	165	19.6	6.4	5.8	—
Halibut						
cooked, broiled	66.6	171	25.2	7.0	0	0
Ice cream and frozen custard						
rich, approximately 16% fat	62.8	222	2.6	16.1	18.0	0
Ice cream cones	8.9	377	10.0	2.4	77.9	.2
Ice milk	66.7	152	4.8	5.1	22.4	0
Ices, water, lime	66.9	78	.4	trace	32.6	trace
Jams and preserves	29.0	272	.6	.1	70.0	1.0

†Sugars, starches, and fiber

Food and Description	Water %	Calories	Protein	Fat	Carbo-hydrate Total†	Fiber Only
Lamb						
composite of cuts						
prime grade						
(72% lean, 28% fat)	56.3	310	15.4	27.1	0	0
choice grade						
cooked, roasted						
(83% lean, 17% fat)	54.0	279	25.3	18.9	0	0
rib						
prime grade						
cooked, broiled						
chops (53% lean,						
47% fat)	35.5	492	16.9	46.5	0	0
Lard	0	902	0	100.0	0	0
Lemons, raw						
peeled fruit	90.1	27	1.1	.3	8.2	.4
Lentils, mature seeds						
cooked	72.0	106	7.8	trace	19.3	1.2
Lettuce, raw						
butter head	95.1	14	1.2	.2	2.5	.5
crisp head	95.5	13	.9	.1	2.9	.5
Limes, acid type, raw	89.3	28	.7	.2	9.5	.5
Liver						
beef						
cooked, fried	56.0	229	26.4	10.6	5.3	0
calf						
cooked, fried	51.4	261	29.5	13.2	4.0	0
Lobster, northern						
canned or cooked	76.8	95	18.7	1.5	.3	—
Lobster newburg	64.0	194	18.5	10.6	5.1	—
Lobster salad	80.3	110	10.1	6.4	2.3	—
Macadamia nuts	3.0	691	7.8	71.6	15.9	2.5
Macaroni						
cooked	72.0	111	3.4	.4	23.0	.1
Macaroni and cheese						
canned	80.2	95	3.9	4.0	10.7	.1
Mackerel						
cooked, broiled	61.6	236	21.8	15.8	0	0
Margarine	15.5	720	.6	81.0	.4	0

†Sugars, starches, and fiber

Food and Description	Water %	Calories	Protein	Fat	Carbo-hydrate Total†	Fiber Only
Milk, cow						
fluid						
whole	87.4	65	3.5	3.5	4.9	0
chocolate, skim milk	82.8	76	3.3	2.3	10.9	trace
hot chocolate	80.5	95	3.3	5.0	10.4	.1
hot cocoa	79.0	97	3.8	4.6	10.9	.1
Mushrooms						
raw	90.4	28	2.7	.3	4.4	.8
canned, solids and						
liquids	93.1	17	1.9	.1	2.4	.6
Muskmelons						
raw						
cantaloupe	91.2	30	.7	.1	7.5	.3
casaba	91.5	27	1.2	trace	6.5	.5
honeydew	90.6	33	.8	.3	7.7	.6
Mustard, prepared						
brown	78.1	91	5.9	6.3	5.3	1.3
yellow	80.2	75	4.7	4.4	6.4	1.0
Oatmeal or rolled oats						
dry form	8.3	390	14.2	7.4	68.2	1.2
cooked	86.5	55	2.0	1.0	9.7	.2
Oils, salad or cooking	0	884	0	100.0	0	0
Olives, pickled, canned						
or bottled						
green	78.2	116	1.4	12.7	1.3	1.3
Onions, mature						
raw	89.1	38	1.5	.1	8.7	.6
cooked, boiled	91.8	29	1.2	.1	6.5	.6
Onions, young green						
bulb and entire top	89.4	36	1.5	.2	8.2	(1.2)
Oranges, raw						
all varieties	86.0	49	1.0	.2	12.2	.5
Orange juice						
all varieties	88.3	45	.7	.2	10.4	.1
Oysters						
raw, meat only						
eastern	84.6	66	8.4	1.8	3.4	—
Pancakes, home recipe						
enriched flour	50.1	231	7.1	7.0	34.1	.1

†Sugars, starches, and fiber

Food and Description	Water %	Calories	Protein	Fat	Carbo-hydrate Total†	Fiber Only
Parsnips						
raw	79.1	76	1.7	.5	17.5	2.0
cooked, boiled	82.2	66	1.5	.5	14.9	2.0
Peaches						
raw	89.1	38	.6	.1	9.7	.6
Peanuts						
roasted and salted	1.6	585	26.0	49.8	18.8	2.4
Peanut butter						
some fat and salt	1.8	581	27.8	49.4	17.2	1.9
Peas, edible podded						
raw	83.3	53	3.4	.2	12.0	1.2
cooked, boiled	86.6	43	2.9	.2	9.5	1.2
Peas, green						
cooked	81.5	71	5.4	.4	12.1	2.0
Peas and carrots, frozen, cooked, boiled	85.8	53	3.2	.3	10.1	1.5
Peppers, sweet						
raw	93.4	22	1.2	.2	4.8	1.4
Pickles						
cucumber, dill	93.3	11	.7	.2	2.2	.5
Pies						
baked						
apple	47.6	256	2.2	11.1	38.1	.4
pecan	19.5	418	5.1	22.9	51.3	.5
Pineapple						
raw	85.3	52	.4	.2	13.7	.4
canned						
water pack	89.1	39	.3	.1	10.2	.3
Pineapple juice						
canned, unsweetened	85.6	55	.4	.1	13.5	.1
Pizza, with cheese						
home recipe	48.3	236	12.0	8.3	28.3	.3
Plums, raw	81.1	66	.5	trace	17.8	.4
Popcorn						
popped						
plain	4.0	386	12.7	5.0	76.7	2.2

†Sugars, starches, and fiber

Food and Description	Water %	Calories	Protein	Fat	Carbo-hydrate Total†	Fiber Only
Pork, fresh						
carcass						
bacon or belly	26.4	631	7.1	66.6	0	0
retail cuts						
ham						
medium fat class						
cooked, roasted						
(74% lean, 26% fat)	45.5	374	23.0	30.6	0	0
dry, long cure						
ham						
lean	49.0	310	19.5	25.0	.3	0
Potatoes						
raw	79.8	76	2.1	.1	17.1	.5
cooked						
baked in skin	75.1	93	2.6	.1	21.1	.6
french fried	44.7	274	4.3	13.2	36.0	1.0
Potato chips	1.8	568	5.3	39.8	50.0	(1.6)
Potato sticks	1.5	544	6.4	36.4	50.8	1.5
Pretzels	4.5	390	9.8	4.5	75.9	.3
Prunes						
cooked						
without sugar	66.4	119	1.0	.3	31.4	.8
Puddings						
chocolate	65.8	148	3.1	4.7	25.7	.2
vanilla	76.0	111	3.5	3.9	15.9	trace
Pumpkin						
raw	91.6	26	1.0	.1	6.5	1.1
Radishes, raw						
common	94.5	17	1.0	.1	3.6	.7
Raisins, natural						
uncooked	18.0	289	2.5	.2	77.4	.9
Raspberries						
raw						
black	80.8	73	1.5	1.4	15.7	5.1
red	84.2	57	1.2	.5	13.6	3.0
Rice						
white						
raw	12.0	363	6.7	.4	80.4	.3
cooked	72.6	109	2.0	.1	24.2	.1

†Sugars, starches, and fiber

Food and Description	Water %	Calories	Protein	Fat	Carbo-hydrate Total†	Fiber Only
Rolls and buns						
hard rolls						
enriched	25.4	312	9.8	3.2	59.5	.2
unenriched	25.4	312	9.8	3.2	59.5	.2
whole wheat rolls	32.0	257	10.0	2.8	52.3	1.6
Salad dressings, commercial						
Blue and						
Roquefort cheese:						
regular	32.3	504	4.8	52.3	7.4	.1
low-calorie:						
low-fat (approx. 5 cal. per tsp.)	83.7	76	3.0	5.9	4.1	.1
low-fat (approx. 1 cal. per tsp.)	93.1	19	1.4	1.1	1.4	.1
French:						
regular	38.8	410	.6	38.9	17.5	.3
low-fat with artificial sweetener (approx. 1 cal. per tsp.)	95.2	10	.4	.2	1.8	.3
Italian:						
regular	27.5	552	.2	60.0	6.9	trace
special dietary (low-cal., approx. 2 cal. per tsp.)	90.1	50	.2	4.7	2.9	trace
Salmon						
Atlantic, canned solids and liquids	64.2	203	21.7	12.2	0	0
Sauerkraut, canned solids and liquids	92.8	18	1.0	.2	4.0	.7
Sausage						
bologna						
all samples	56.2	304	12.1	27.5	1.1	—
frankfurters						
all meat	56.5	296	13.1	25.5	2.5	0
pork sausage						
cooked	34.8	476	18.1	44.2	trace	0
salami						
dry	29.8	450	23.8	38.1	1.2	0

†Sugars, starches, and fiber

Food and Description	Water %	Calories	Protein	Fat	Carbo-hydrate Total†	Fiber Only
Scallops						
raw	79.8	81	15.3	.2	3.3	—
cooked, steamed	73.1	112	23.2	1.4	—	—
frozen, breaded, fried						
reheated	60.2	194	18.0	8.4	10.5	—
Sherbet, orange	67.0	134	.9	1.2	30.8	0
Shrimp						
raw	78.2	91	18.1	.8	1.5	—
Soups, commercial						
canned						
chicken noodle						
condensed	86.6	53	2.8	1.6	6.6	.1
chicken rice						
condensed	89.6	39	2.6	1.0	4.7	.1
onion						
condensed	86.9	54	4.4	2.1	4.3	.4
Spaghetti						
enriched						
cooked, tender	72.0	111	3.4	.4	23.0	.1
Spaghetti with meatballs						
in tomato sauce						
canned	78.0	134	7.5	4.7	15.6	.3
Spanish, mackerel, raw	68.9	177	19.5	10.4	0	0
Spanish rice						
home recipe	78.5	87	1.8	1.7	16.6	.5
Spinach						
raw	90.7	26	3.2	.3	4.3	.6
cooked, boiled	92.0	23	3.0	.3	3.6	.6
Squash						
summer						
all varieties						
raw	94.0	19	1.1	.1	4.2	.6
cooked, boiled	95.5	14	.9	.1	3.1	.6
winter						
cooked, baked	81.4	63	1.8	.4	15.4	1.8
acorn						
boiled, mashed	89.7	34	1.2	.1	8.4	1.4
Strawberries						
raw	89.9	37	.7	.5	8.4	1.3

†Sugars, starches, and fiber

Food and Description	Water %	Calories	Protein	Fat	Carbo-hydrate Total†	Fiber Only
Succotash (corn and lima beans), frozen cooked, boiled	74.1	93	4.2	.4	20.5	.9
Sugars powdered	.5	385	0	0	99.5	0
Swordfish raw	75.9	118	19.2	4.0	0	0
cooked, broiled	64.6	174	28.0	6.0	0	0
canned, liquids and solids	78.0	102	17.5	3.0	0	0
Tartar sauce regular	34.4	531	1.4	57.8	4.2	.3
Tomatoes, ripe raw	93.5	22	1.1	.2	4.7	.5
cooked, boiled	92.4	26	1.3	.2	5.5	.6
Tomato catsup, bottled	68.6	106	2.0	.4	25.4	.5
Tomato chili sauce, bottled	68.0	104	2.5	.3	24.8	.7
Tomato juice canned or bottled regular pack	93.6	19	.9	.1	4.3	.2
special dietary pack (low sodium)	94.2	19	.8	.1	4.3	.2
Tuna canned in oil	52.6	288	24.2	20.5	0	0
Tuna salad	69.8	170	14.6	10.5	3.5	—
Turkey flesh only cooked, roasted	61.2	190	31.5	6.1	0	0
light meat cooked, roasted	62.1	176	32.9	3.9	0	0
dark meat cooked, roasted	60.5	203	30.0	8.3	0	0
Turnips cooked, boiled	93.6	23	.8	.2	4.9	.9
Veal thin class (88% lean 12% fat)	71.0	156	19.7	8.0	0	0

†Sugars, starches, and fiber

Food and Description	Water %	Calories	Protein	Fat	Carbo-hydrate Total†	Fiber Only
Veal cont'd						
flank						
thin class						
total edible, raw						
(73% lean, 27% fat)	63.0	240	18.1	18.0	0	0
Vegetable juice cocktail						
canned	94.1	17	.9	.1	3.6	.3
Vinegar						
cider	93.8	14	trace	*	5.9	—
Waffles						
baked, home recipe	41.4	279	9.3	9.8	37.5	.1
Walnuts						
black	3.1	628	20.5	59.3	14.8	1.7
Watermelon						
raw	92.6	26	.5	.2	6.4	.3
Yogurt						
skim milk	89.0	50	3.4	1.7	5.2	0
whole milk	88.0	62	3.0	3.4	4.9	0

†Sugars, starches, and fiber
*Too low to measure.

AMOUNT OF CHOLESTEROL IN 100 GRAMS
(EDIBLE PORTION) EXPRESSED IN MILLIGRAMS

Beef, raw		Lamb, raw	
with bone	70	with bone	70
without bone	70	without bone	70
Brains, raw greater than 2,000		Lard and other animal fat	95
Butter	250	Liver, raw	300
Caviar or fish roe greater than 300		Lobster	
Cheese		whole	200
Cheddar	100	meat only	200
Cottage, creamed	15	Margarine	
Cream	120	all vegetable fat	0
Other (25% to 30% fat)	85	⅔ animal fat, ⅓ vegetable fat	65
Cheese spread	65	Milk	
Chicken, flesh only, raw	60	fluid, whole	11
Crab		dried, whole	85
in shell	125	fluid, skim	3
meat only	125	Oysters	
Egg, whole	550	in shell greater than 200	
Egg white	0	meat only greater than 200	
Egg yolk		Pork	
fresh	1,500	with bone	70
frozen	1,280	without bone	70
dried	2,950	Shrimp	
Fish		in shell	125
steak	70	flesh only	125
fillet	70	Sweetbreads (thymus)	250
Heart, raw	150	Veal	
Ice cream	45	with bone	90
Kidney, raw	375	without bone	90

Index